A Desire to Help

Most people develop a determination to see that their children have better lives than what they, themselves, experienced. Brenda (Susie) Hutchings was born with a desire to be an influence on producing good outcomes in healthful living for those she encounters – particularly the elderly.

Such a heart filled with compassion drove her to earn a bachelor of science degree in nursing at East Tennessee State University in Johnson City, the same institution where she is now working toward a master of public health degree. She is also Certified in Gerontology (RN, C), is a licensed nursing home administrator and is certified as a professional in health care quality (CPHQ).

Hutchings has more than 20 years in acute and long-term care nursing administration and operations. She has extensive experience in quality assurance, Alzheimer's work, drug utilization and skilled care programs. She began her nursing career at Unicoi County Memorial Hospital in Erwin, Tennessee, as a staff nurse, progressing to charge nurse, in-service director and to director of quality assurance.

In 1984, she joined Life Care Centers of America as director of nursing at its Erwin facility, and advanced to her present position as senior vice president of clinical services. Along the way, she has won many professional honors, including director of nursing of the year in Tennessee in 1989-90 and the Tennessee Health Care Association's Distinguished Professional Service Award in 1991.

Hutchings has authored a number of publications and papers, and has done numerous presentations to national organizations on Alzheimer's disease, conflict management, quality assurance and staff management. Among her many accomplishments are:

- Development of a facility quality assurance program adopted in many nursing centers throughout the United States.
- Implementation of a facility drug utilization program that received national recognition, including a presentation before the U.S. Special Senate Committee on Aging in Washington, D.C.
- Establishment of a state-approved training program for certified nursing assistants.

On the personal side, Hutchings and her husband, Jeff, have three daughters: Ginger and Gretchen Hutchings, and Mrs. Bryan (Gennie) Edwards.

THEY CALL IT LOVE

by

Brenda "Susie" Hutchings

FOREWORD

People who achieve greatness in their lives have a passion for what they do. They are driven by an incessant, burning desire to find a new product or to create an avenue of service that enhances the journey of us all. They distinguish themselves by what they do with what they find in everyday experiences.

Brenda (or Susie, as I know her) Hutchings is one of the truly great individuals I have had the privilege of knowing. If greatness is measured by accomplishment in the political realm or in the entertainment business, arenas where the word is most overused... well, that's not Hutchings. But if it is assessed in terms of enrichment of the quality of life – the imprints for good that can be made on the slate of human existence – then it is an apt description of her.

Hutchings' singular goal in life, often whispered in prayer-like fashion when confronted with a difficult circumstance or situation, is: "If I can just make a difference in one person's life...."

Time after time, she does. The truth is, she makes substantial contributions to many. Everyday.

This book is the realization of a longtime dream. A former director of nursing and now senior vice president of clinical services for Life Care Centers of America, Hutchings carries a heavy burden for those who fill the role of directing the care in a nursing facility. "They Call It Love" is written for the D.O.N. and anyone who aspires to be. It offers excellent advice on organization of responsibilities, development of systems and procedures, building the team and interaction with residents and families. As with any counsel that flows from Hutchings, this publication is a blending of the mind and the heart, to the benefit of both body and soul, couched in the Christian ethic.

The author recognizes the frustrations and anxieties of the director of nursing, and she gives hope and reassurance, along with valuable information, thereby instilling confidence, for the important work that is to be done.

"They Call It Love" is also recommended reading for anyone in long-term health care who needs the perspective of this pivotal, and demanding, position of leadership in a nursing facility.

Beecher Hunter
Executive Vice President
Life Care Centers of America

Acknowledgements

This is a first! I never really dreamed that, some day, I would write a book. I suppose it is normal to feel a sense of gratitude to a few people at a time such as this in one's life. Where do I begin? How do I say "thank you" to those who have been a significant part of my life?

My parents, Thelma and Luther Wilkinson, taught me the importance of, and instilled in me the desire, to be the best that I could be. I was taught from a very early age that there is a Master and a Master plan, and that my role in life was to give of my best to the Master.

My husband, Geoffrey, and my daughters, Gennifer, Gretchen and Ginger, have been very encouraging and supportive of my work since they, also, understand the importance of the Master's plan.

There have been many others who have supported, encouraged and taught me throughout my career. Not long ago, my husband gave to me a plaque that says, "Every experience God gives us. Every person He puts in our lives, is the perfect preparation for the future that only He can see."

He has certainly placed many very special people in my life for whom I am very thankful.

Brenda "Susie" Hutchings

1

Philosophy

Basically, I believe that we must have a genuine concern, compassion and respect for all of those around us. We must strive to constantly maintain this philosophy in dealing with residents, family members and associates. We must support one another consistently and look for the good in each other. We must see through the eyes of God's love. Love is the motivational force that has no match. It is the magic ingredient causing people to "want to" do that which is right.

We must provide an atmosphere in which the people are allowed to learn to grow and to improve without the constant fear of being disciplined in a way that would be degrading. In this atmosphere we can provide the opportunity for the weaknesses, which we and all of our associates have, to become our strengths. Teaching is an important part of this philosophy. Remember that "the teacher has taught when the student has learned." To tell someone how to perform a particular task is only a very small part of teaching. The individual has been taught only when he/she can demonstrate the ability to perform in accordance with instruction.

By providing this environment for all of our associates, and by readily accepting change, every associate is allowed to learn, grow and become the best person he/she can be. These procedures will allow the entire facility to become the best that it can be.

Management Concepts

TRUTH–*the quality or state of being true and in conformity with the facts. Search for the facts in order to get to the truth in any situation. Accept no accusations and get all the facts before assessing the problem and making a decision of any kind, including discipline, specific changes in policy, procedural changes and developing strategic plans.*

HONESTY–*refraining from lying, cheating or stealing: being trustworthy and upright. Tell your associates the truth and do not make promises you cannot keep or that are outside of your authority to grant. Teach them to trust you.*

JUSTICE–*impartiality and fairness. Give rewards or penalties as deserved. Treat all associates and others equally. Be fair and consistent.*

PURE–*free from defects; perfect, faultless. Live so that your associates and others see in you an example worth following.*

LOVELY–*having those qualities that inspire love, affection and admiration. Look for these qualities in your associates and others to bring these attributes to the surface and submerge those which are not desirable.*

VIRTUE–*goodness and excellence. Work continuously toward excellence by doing that which is good.*

PRAISE–*to commend the worth of; to express approval or admiration of. Always praise your associates when they do a job well.*

"Finally brethren, whatsoever things are honest, whatsoever things are just, whatsoever things are pure, whatsoever things are lovely, whatsoever things are of good report: if there be any virtue, and if there be any praise, think on these things."

Philippians 4:8

LOVE

If I could explain everything to my associates but did not LOVE each one of them, I might as well be talking to an empty room.

If I had all of the answers to the regulatory legal and ethical issues and did not have LOVE, my efforts would be futile.

If I had an abundance of supplies and personnel and personally sacrificed to do so but did not have LOVE for those around me, it would be a complete waste.

LOVE is patient when it is necessary to teach repeatedly the new concept to those around us.

LOVE is kind when an irate patient accuses and berates others or me.

LOVE is not jealous when I am pleased with the accomplishments of others.

LOVE is not proud and boastful when my staff produces positive results, but I instead am humble and thankful.

LOVE is being willing to yield my schedule and plans to fit the needs of others.

LOVE does not demand that others comply with my rules, but seeks to help them to understand the importance of self-discipline.

LOVE does not tell of others' shortcomings to those around me.

LOVE keeps trying even when it seems that no one understands my purpose and my mission.

Theories, concepts, memos and textbooks will eventually be discarded, but LOVE is everlasting.

These three things I have learned: endurance, patience and LOVE, but the greatest of these is LOVE.

INTRODUCTION

With the increase in the elderly population, it will continue to be necessary for the long-term care industry to produce a quality of care which in turn will produce a quality of life.

This book has been written primarily for directors of nursing in long term care facilities. It is designed to help them understand how to better organize and administer the duties of that office as well as to help them deal with the emotional impact of their environment.

The concepts expressed by the words Leadership, Oneness, Values *and* Empowerment *are those that will help each of us manage our facilities more efficiently so as to provide the superior quality of care we are striving to achieve.*

As directors of nursing we learn that leadership does not involve giving direct patient care ourselves, but the enlisting and training of others to perform these tasks. As we carefully supervise the performance of our associates, we assure that proper care is being provided. Oneness is defined as a common goal or a common purpose. Our number one priority is to work together to produce a superior quality of care for our residents. Each of us individually must assess our value system and "do what we value and value what we do." Empowerment is the enabling of those we lead to use their abilities in such a way that they become the best that they can be.

My hope in publishing this book is that some day the director of nursing of a long-term care facility will say, "I am proud to be a long-term care nurse."

THEY CALL IT...

LEADERSHIP

ONENESS

VALUES

EMPOWERMENT

TABLE OF CONTENTS

SECTION I ADMINISTRATION

SECTION II PATIENT CARE

SECTION III QUALITY ASSURANCE

SECTION I

ADMINISTRATION

CHAPTER I

THE STANDARD OF CARE

Nursing is a very special profession; a profession that requires the combined effort of every emotional feeling, every physical sense and every mental capability that a person has. The challenge is great, the opportunities are never-ending and the rewards are incredible. How do you describe the feelings that evolve as you care for another human being? The range of emotions from love to hate, peace to anger, from freedom to total fear of movement can be expressed and sometimes felt going from one extreme end of the spectrum to the other in the blink of an eye.

Nurses can operate the most intricate machinery, tabulate the appropriate information from detailed scientific and mathematical equations under extremely stressful situations, and yet can have the capacity and take the time to touch, hold, love and care about the person to whom they minister.

When I became a registered nurse, I felt that my ultimate goal, dream and vision of a lifetime had been accomplished. Little did I realize that it was only the beginning—the beginning of learning, growing and teaching in the form of a continuous ongoing cycle. As I progressed through that cycle, I eventually became the director of nursing of a long-term care facility. Again, it became evident that this was a new beginning—a new opportunity to learn, grow and teach.

As I entered into my new role as director of nursing, I realized that one of the first items for consideration was the establishment of nursing standards in this environment. The questions began to emerge. What was the standard of care to which we would aspire and maintain in this facility? I remember the knot in my stomach and the lump in my throat as I fought the battle within myself over the standard that I felt should be maintained. At the same time, I envisioned the very practical components that would make that standard a difficult task to attain—the issues of funding and staffing.

After much thought and deliberation, I finally realized that the vision of the standard of care I desired and the anticipation of attaining that standard would be the driving forces to make it happen. One truth I learned as a manager is that I, as well as those around me, must live up to the expected standard of care.

The specific standards of care established at that point in time were:

1. **Staffing**

   Individual nursing care assignments shall be based upon patient need, skill levels and individual personnel ability.

2. **Communication**

   Nursing personnel will communicate with physicians to assure maximum interpretation and processing of diagnostic and therapeutic orders given for patient care and to provide for their implementation and coordination.

3. **Patient Care**

   Nursing personnel will administer appropriate medications, provide all treatments and, in general, assure the best possible patient outcomes.

4. **Confidentiality**

   All information received from or about a resident and/or facility personnel will be shared only with appropriate facility personnel or other authorized individuals for the benefit of the individual and/or facility involved.

5. **Discharge Planning**

   Each resident shall be evaluated on an ongoing basis to determine discharge status and should be encouraged and assisted to return home if at all possible.

6. **Patient Education**

   Nursing personnel will instruct patients and/or families as necessary concerning treatments, conditions and medications in keeping with professional and legal guidelines.

7. **Records/Reports**

   All nursing written records, care plans and reports will be maintained in accordance with facility policies and procedures.

8. **Infection Control**

   Nursing personnel will adhere to all infection control guidelines.

9. **Safety**

   Nursing personnel shall be able to recognize possible safety hazards and demonstrate proper protocol to follow in the event of such hazards.

10. **Orientation**

    All nursing personnel or volunteers will have complete orientation to the facility and appropriate policies and procedures.

Once the standards were established, the questions began to evolve. How do I attain these standards and how do I maintain them? One very significant point that quickly became evident to me is the importance of involving every member of my staff in the development and implementation of these standards. Valuable results are obtained by discussing the standards with the entire staff in small group meetings in order to provide opportunity for free discussion and "brainstorming." One way to accomplish this is to meet first with the registered nurses and licensed practical nurses and then with the nursing assistants per shift per month. I have also learned that we may know what all of the answers are, but do we know what questions will stimulate conversation to the end that everyone collectively might decide what the answers will be?

Let's look at each of the standards and determine what some of the questions may be.

STAFFING

1. What are the needs of our patients?
2. What kind of knowledge base does our staff have?
3. Have we identified the needs of our patients that the staff is not equipped with knowledge or skills to meet?
4. Do we need to educate our staff?
5. Do we need to improve the organization of our staff?

COMMUNICATION

1. What do we need to communicate to physicians?
2. What do we need to communicate regarding implementation and coordination?
3. With whom do we need to communicate regarding implementation and coordination?
4. What procedures need to be put into place in order to adequately communicate regarding implementation and coordination?

PATIENT CARE

1. What are the ten most common medications administered in the facility?
2. Are the nurses knowledgeable concerning the reasons for, side effects, etc., of those medications?
3. What time of day is the medication administered?
4. Could the times of administration be more efficiently organized?
5. What kind of lab work is required routinely because of those medications?
6. What kind of treatments are necessary for our patients?
7. How do we provide for the activities of daily living for our patients?
8. What are the top 25 quality of care indicators that we should consistently monitor?

CONFIDENTIALITY

1. How do we ensure that confidentiality is being maintained among ourselves and our residents?

DISCHARGE PLANNING

1. Do we evaluate our patients upon admission for the potential of discharge from the facility?
2. Do we keep records of those who have the potential to be discharged at this point in time in our facility?
3. Do we have procedures in place to prepare residents and families for that discharge?

PATIENT EDUCATION

1. Do our patients or other designated persons know about their plan of care?
2. Do our patients or other designated persons know their rights?

RECORDS AND REPORTS

1. Do we have appropriate documentation in place to assure continuity of care?

INFECTION CONTROL

1. Are we aware, on a daily basis, of each resident in the facility who has an infection?
2. Are we reviewing all infections on at least a monthly basis to identify trends and consistently improve negative trends on an ongoing basis?

SAFETY

1. Are we aware, on a daily basis, of all accident incidents of associates/patients?
2. Do we evaluate all incidents on a monthly basis to identify specific trends and continuously improve our process?

ORIENTATION

1. What kind of associate orientation program do we have?
2. Are we confident that our associates are able to complete their job duties once they have completed that orientation program?

Once these questions are asked and answered, and as our associates realize that we do have an established standard of care that is expected to be maintained, they will begin to live up to that expectation.

EXCELLENCE

Excellence can be attained if you...

Care more than others think is wise.

Risk more than others think is safe.

Dream more than others think is practical.

Expect more than others think is possible.

CHAPTER II

ADMINISTRATIVE POLICY

Nursing administration is certainly a challenge to anyone. One of the most amazing discoveries to me was the fact that by being a staff nurse, I thought I knew all of the answers regarding administration. When I became a nursing administrator, I suddenly realized I had forgotten those answers. I found myself asking questions such as: Why is being a nurse manager so difficult? Why is it so hard for us to separate doing and managing? Words such as planning, organizing, delegating, controlling, etc., began to come to mind—words that I was not very comfortable with at that point in time. Nurses are not trained to delegate; they are trained to do.

I realized that day by day I was not very successfully "crisis managing" my facility. All day long I was putting out fires, fighting battle after battle, only to find more fires to put out and more battles to be fought the following day. This did not produce quality patient care and it certainly was a frustrating experience. This was only day-to-day survival.

I remember attending one of my daughter's band concerts one evening. As I watched the band perform, an interesting observation occurred. What was the band director doing? He was directing the band. If he had chosen to play the flute, the drums or the saxophone at any given point, I believe the band could have made mistakes for lack of direction. I viewed that scenario as applicable to what I should be doing as a director of nursing. I needed to direct, not crisis-manage given sections of the nursing department on a day-to-day basis, but orchestrate the total nursing department on a broader, ongoing scale.

The next step in the process of implementing a formalized management structure was to develop and carry out nursing administrative policies.

The nursing department shall be under the full-time supervision of a registered professional nurse who is currently licensed by the state. The director of nursing shall have one year of education and/or experience in nursing service administration. The director should also have education and/or experience in such areas as rehabilitative, psychiatric and/or gerontological nursing. The director shall attend continuing education programs at least annually and this course of action shall be at least annually and this course of action shall be fully documented. The director of nursing shall be employed on a full-time basis.

The director of nursing shall be directly responsible to the executive director. The director shall be responsible for and accountable to the executive director for the functions and activities of the nursing staff. In the absence of the director of nursing, responsibility for continuity and supervision of nursing care shall be delegated to a qualified individual.

All nursing individuals shall be fully licensed by the state or shall have a current temporary license with a stated expiration date. The director of nursing shall verify every nursing license by initially establishing:

1. Identity of the person.
2. Presentation of the license and annual renewal of such license, transcribing and keeping on file the renewal number.
3. No copy of a license, renewal certificate or permit belonging to an individual may be made.
4. No photostatic copy for identification will be accepted.
5. A current renewal certificate must be reviewed, the individual's name, license number, and expiration date recorded and recognized as an official document.

The director of nursing shall be responsible for:

1. Developing and maintaining nursing service philosophy, objectives, standards of practice, policy and procedure manuals and job descriptions for each level of nursing personnel.
2. Recommending to the executive director the number and level of nursing personnel to be employed.
3. Employing nursing personnel, including their recruitment, selection, position assignment, orientation and in-service education, supervision, evaluation and termination.
4. Participating with the executive director and medical director in the allocation of funds for facility programs.
5. Participating with the medical director and executive director in developing and implementing patient care policies.
6. Assuring that a current plan of care is maintained for each patient in conjunction with other disciplines required to provide total care.
7. Evaluating nursing care.
8. Coordinating nursing services with other services, such as medical services, physical and occupational therapy, social services,

dietary services, the patient activity program and the scheduling of rounds to see patients.

The director of nursing shall designate a charge nurse for each shift who shall be responsible for the supervision of all nursing activities in the facility or in the section to which he/she is assigned.

1. The charge nurse shall be either a currently licensed practical nurse who has experience in nursing service, supervision and training and/or experience in rehabilitative, psychiatric and/or gerontological nursing.

2. The charge nurse on each shift shall be responsible for (a) making daily patient visits to assess physical and emotional status of the patient and implementing any required nursing interventions, (b) reviewing medication records for completeness of information, accuracy in the transcription of physician orders and adherence to stop-order policies, (c) assigning responsibility for direct patient care to the nursing staff, (d) supervising and evaluating performance of all nursing personnel on the unit and (e) keeping the director of nursing informed of the status of patients and other related matters.

The facility shall provide 24-hour nursing care services to meet the nursing needs of all patients. There shall be a registered nurse assigned eight hours per day, seven days per week.

There shall be a licensed practical nurse assigned to each shift seven days a week. Currently licensed practical nurses, certified nursing assistants shall be assigned duties consistent with their education and/or experience. Sufficient nursing personnel shall be assigned and on duty to assure that the following conditions are met:

1. Patients are provided safe and efficient nursing care.
2. Patients receive all treatments, medications and diets as prescribed.
3. Patients are provided rehabilitative nursing care as needed.
4. Patients are provided proper care to prevent pressure ulcers and deformities.
5. Patients are kept comfortable, clean, neat, well groomed and protected from accident, injury or infection.
6. Patients are encouraged, assisted and trained in self care.

Time schedules indicating the number and classification of nursing personnel, including relief personnel, shall be maintained and posted on each unit at least one week in advance. Schedule changes indicating who worked on each unit for every shift shall be documented and maintained on file.

All medications for patients shall be prescribed by a licensed physician. All prescriptions are to be dispersed in accordance with written drug orders. All verbal drug orders shall be given to a licensed nurse by the physician. These orders shall be signed by the accepting person and countersigned by the attending physician within 48 hours.

The physician, pharmacist and charge nurse shall review each patient's medications on a monthly basis or whenever there is a change in the patient's condition. Orders for medications shall be renewed by a physician's signature every 30 days. The following policies concerning stop orders on potent drugs must be carried out:

1. All orders for drugs, including prn orders, should be written for a specific period of time or an exact number of doses.
2. When no time or dose limitations are specified on the original order, automatic stop orders on all drugs will be effective as follows: (a) all scheduled III and IV drugs and anticoagulants will carry a 30-day stop order, (b) antibiotics will be discontinued in seven days, (c) all scheduled II drugs shall have a 72-hour stop order.

3. When a drug needs to be reordered or stopped, the nursing personnel will verbally notify the attending physician that a new order is needed. If the order expires in the night, it should be called to the attention of the physician the following morning. All drugs and biologicals shall be stored under proper conditions of temperature, light and security. Medications shall be stored in a well-illuminated, locked storage cabinet, and shall be accessible only to authorized personnel—director of nursing, charge nurse, pharmacist or medication nurse.

Medications being distributed shall be kept under continuous supervision. Medications for external use only shall be stored separately from internal medications and shall be accessible only to authorized personnel. Schedule II controlled drugs shall be stored in a cabinet of substantial construction under a double lock system.

The medications for each patient shall be stored in original containers and shall not be transferred to other containers for storage. Each patient's medication shall be kept separate from others. With the exception of unit dose packages, each original container shall be legibly marked with a securely attached label that clearly indicates the patient's full name, physician's name, prescription number, instruction for administration, date received, expiration date of all time-dated drugs, and the name, address and telephone number of the pharmacy issuing the drug. Medication containers that are damaged or poorly labeled shall be returned to the pharmacy for relabeling or disposal.

Pharmaceuticals requiring refrigeration shall be stored in a refrigerator located in a locked area. The temperature of the refrigerator shall be checked every day.

Medications shall be administered only by physicians or licensed nursing personnel. Medications are to be administered as soon as possible after doses are prepared and are to be administered by the same person who prepared the dose. Each medication administered and the time of administration shall be promptly recorded in the patient's individual medication record and signed with the first and last name and position of the individual who administered the medication.

Medications prescribed for one patient shall not be administered to any other patient. Self administration of medications by patients shall be permitted only when specially authorized in writing by the attending physician. Control and supervision, however, is still the responsibility of the facility.

Medication errors and adverse reactions shall be reported to the patient's physician, the nursing supervisor and the pharmacist. If the situation is potentially life-threatening, it shall be reported immediately. All medication errors shall be filed as an incident and reported to the director of nursing.

For control of Schedule II drugs, a separate record listing the following information shall be maintained for each substance:

1. Substance
2. Prescription
3. Amount received
4. Patient's name
5. Date and time administered
6. Dose
7. Physician's name
8. Signature of person administering the drug
9. Balance remaining

Records of controlled drugs are to be maintained in sufficient detail for accurate reconciliation. A count of narcotics shall be documented and signed at the end of each shift by the individual responsible.

Drugs are to be checked monthly for expiration date. If the drug is outdated, it shall be reported to the pharmacist who shall prevent distribution and administration. Any patient-requisitioned drug that is not used must be returned to the pharmacy when the patient is discharged unless the physician requests that the patient take the medication home. Any drug that is discontinued is returned immediately to the pharmacy. Credit will be issued only on unit dose or unit of medication. All other medications shall be destroyed.

In the event of a drug recall, each nursing station is contacted either by telephone or in person and instructed to return the recall drug to the pharmacy for credit. The pharmacy shall serve as a drug information center.

Each resident shall be assessed according to the Resident Assessment Instrument (RAI) process.

A written nursing care plan shall be initiated and maintained for each patient based on the nature of the illness, treatment prescribed, long- and short-term goals and other pertinent information. The nursing care plan will be a personalized plan for individual patients. It will indicate that nursing care is needed, the way in which it can best be accomplished for each patient, how a patient likes to have things done, what methods and approaches are most successful and what modifications are necessary to ensure the best results. A plan of care shall be developed by the following personnel: (a) nurses, (b) dietitians, (c) activity directors, (d) physical therapists, (e) social service agents and other responsible individuals. This plan of care, including the assessment of the total needs of the patient, and the development of care plans to meet those needs shall be completed within the first 21 days of stay and re-evaluated every three months. The plan of care shall be available for use by all personnel caring for the patient. Each service may maintain pertinent sections of the plan of care; overall coordination and maintenance of the plan shall be the responsibility of the nursing service. The patient's family or other responsible person(s) shall be aware of the goals of care and should participate in the development and review of the plan.

Dietary supervision shall be provided by nursing personnel. Awareness of the dietary needs and food and fluid intake of the patient will be indicated by: (a) valid evidence that patients are served diets as prescribed, (b) consistent observation of food and fluid intake and sufficient notation of such in the medical record, (c) prompt designation of personnel to assist those who need help with eating, (d) provision of adaptive self-help devices to contribute to the patient's independence in eating, (e) responsible reporting of deviations from normal to the charge nurse and persistent unresolved problems to the physician. The director of nursing or the charge nurse shall coordinate the resolution of patient nutritional problems observed by nursing personnel and report such to the dietitian.

At least three meals or their equivalent shall be served daily, at regular times, with not more than a 14-hour span between a substantial evening meal and breakfast. Bedtime snacks of nourishing quality shall be offered if permitted by the physician in charge. The dietitian shall calculate calories and assess the nutritional status of patients on tube feedings and consult with physicians and nursing staff concerning these items. The dietary supervisor shall visit patients daily to ensure proper dietary care and maintain the nutritional status of each patient.

The facility shall maintain an active program of rehabilitative nursing care to assist each patient in achieving and maintaining an optimum level of functioning and independence through education and training. Rehabilitative nursing services shall be performed daily for all patients who require such services and documentation of services provided. The nursing personnel responsible for providing rehabilitative services shall have received special instruction in rehabilitative techniques, including demonstration, supervision and evaluation.

Written nursing care policies and procedures essential to assure consistency of care and patient safety shall be available for ready reference by all nursing personnel and other involved staff members. These policies and procedures shall be reviewed at least annually and revised as necessary.

Orientation of new personnel shall be conducted by the in-service director. The material covered shall include job descriptions, responsibilities and duties, patient care policies, personnel policies, administrative policies, procedure manuals, a fire and mass casualty plan and a plan of infection control. There shall be an ongoing documented in-service education program for all nursing personnel. The director of nursing shall be responsible for assuring that a review and evaluation of the quality and appropriateness of nursing care is accomplished in a timely manner.

WE MUST FIGHT
TO WIN THE WAR,
NOT JUST THE BATTLE

CHAPTER III

TRAINING AND EDUCATION

Teaching is a very important part of our profession. The empowerment to accomplish our task is, in essence, teaching. We are successful in this or any other profession only to the degree in which we are able to envision every experience we have as either a teaching or learning experience.

Just imagine, if you will, that each time our associates do not meet our standard of performance we are able to see that as an opportunity to teach rather than one to condemn and complain about. If we see every experience of life as a learning adventure, the worst case scenario will help us learn from our mistakes and the best case scenario will challenge us to continuously improve our performance.

Basically, I believe that 99 percent of our associates want to do a good job. The reason people do not meet the established standards or fail to live up to our expectations is a result of one or more of the following: (a) they have a lack of knowledge, (b) they lack the proper skills, (c) they are unable to manage their time effectively, and/or (d) they are unable to prioritize.

This philosophy assists us in categorizing the solutions to our problems. These are the subjects we can teach. Do our associates need more education and training relating to specific procedures or skills? Should we assist them in their endeavor to better manage their time? Remember that we help them prioritize each day by showing them what is important in the overall care of our patients. If it is important to us, it is also important to them. The only time this philosophy does not produce a desired result is if the associate simply does not "want to," but I believe this is the exception—not the rule.

The definition of teaching is:
"To give instruction, to impart knowledge, to cause to learn."

Teaching is so much more than simply telling someone something. In fact, to tell someone something is a very small part of the process. The Tennessee Instructional Model (TIM) tells us that in order to teach we must complete the following steps:

I tell you
You tell me
I show you
You show me.

As we complete this process it becomes evident to the teacher and the student that learning has taken place. The more we teach and learn on a daily basis, the stronger and more effective our facility will be.

It is very important to realize that each of us is a teacher. Maybe we are a teacher because we are giving instruction to our peers. Perhaps we are teaching as we show our associates a new procedure or persuade our boss that a new policy, a new procedure or the establishment of a new staff position is necessary. Teaching is something we can learn to do, thereby changing our entire perspective in dealing with problems and challenges facing us each day.

We must maintain an environment conducive to teaching and be constantly aware of all teaching opportunities that cross our path daily. In this environment people can comfortably say, "I don't know," and this is the point at which learning can take place. As we learn and grow together, our total facility personnel will be able to provide quality care for all of our residents.

Perhaps an appropriate question at this point is, "Why do people learn?" I believe the greatest motivation in the world for teaching is loving and respecting those we teach. If we love, respect and believe in our associates, they will do their best to live up to our expectations. They will "want to" learn. Have you ever learned or accomplished something new because you knew that someone believed in you? Have you ever had an associate come to you and say, "I did not think I could do it, but I knew that you believed that I could?" We all need that kind of support, encouragement, and motivation in order to learn and grow.

My father was a teacher for many years. His motto was, "The teacher has taught when the student has learned." I believe this puts the responsibility for learning where it belongs—with the teacher. There are no excuses. If the teacher is to produce the desired results, he/she must ask the questions: (a) how can I determine what is necessary to motivate the student to learn; and (b) how can I ensure understanding on the part of the student? If this atmosphere prevails, a knowledgeable and skilled work force will emerge that is second to none.

THE TEACHER HAS TAUGHT
WHEN THE STUDENT
HAS LEARNED

CHAPTER IV

STAFFING

One of the greatest challenges for the director of nursing of a long-term care facility is staffing. This challenge very definitely requires the "patience of Job, the wisdom of Solomon, and the love and compassion of Christ." Not that I could attain any of the three, but they certainly are goals to strive for.

Upon initially surveying the staffing issue, we discover there are more questions than answers. When do I hire someone? What should be the process for hiring someone? How many licensed nurses do I need? How many nursing assistants do I need? How do I approach administration regarding staffing? How do I orient my staff? How do I set up an in-service program?

Perhaps the very first question we need to ask is, "What are the budgeted hours per patient day in nursing for our facility?" The executive director can answer that question. Each facility is significantly different in staffing needs. There are many variables; the acuity level of the residents and the educational level of the staff are two important items to consider. Don't make the mistake of comparing staffing requirements with those of another facility. We must evaluate our own needs on an ongoing basis and meet them.

Let's suppose that the budgeted staffing per patient day in a facility is 2.32 hours per patient day. What does that mean? In order to determine how many staff members are included in the budget on any given day, the following equation needs to be applied:

120 patients (total population of the facility)
x 2.32 hours per patient day
278.40 hours (patient care hours per day provided in the facility)
278.40 hours divided by 8 (hours worked per associate)
= 34.8 associates per 24-hour period of time or 35 associates.

The next question to consider is, "How many of those associates should be certified nursing assistants and how many should be licensed personnel?" A good place to begin is to consider 70 percent for certified nursing assistants and 30 percent for licensed nurses. This is not a hard and fast rule but only a beginning point. We need to determine what that percentage would give us to work with, consider the acuity level of the residents, the layout of the facility and then decide what works best.

As we continue, we need to ask how many personnel will be needed on each shift. A good rule to follow is 47 percent of the staffing is required for the day shift, 34 percent for the second shift, and 19 percent for the night shift. Suppose our staffing needs call for a total of 30 certified nursing assistants in a 24-hour period. The day shift would require 47 percent of 30, or a total of 14 certified nursing assistants. The second shift would need 34 percent of 30, or a total of 10 certified nursing assistants for the night shift, 19 percent of 30, or a total of six certified nursing assistants.

Once we determine the number of personnel, we must decide how many associates are required per shift in order to fulfill our staffing levels in the facility. The following table demonstrates the process of making sure that an adequate number of personnel is available to maintain staffing.

Day shift on the south wing—4 CNAs are needed to cover that wing for that shift. To cover that shift for seven days each week would require 4 times 7 or 28 positions to be filled.

To determine if you have enough personnel to fill those positions, list the associates whom you presently have in the following way:

Associate	Number of shifts each works
1. Jane Doe	Five shifts per week
2. John Brown	Five shifts per week
3. Sally Smith	Five shifts per week, etc.

15 shifts per week are covered Further, 28 minus 15 equals 13 shifts per week that are not covered. Therefore, you need two full-time associates at five days per week and one part-time associate at three days per week to completely staff that shift.

The sum total of the number of shifts worked must equal the total number of shifts needed to be covered for the entire week. By reviewing each shift in this way, we can determine whether or not we have adequate staffing and if we should hire additional personnel.

It cannot be emphasized enough how important it is to apply this methodology in determining staffing needs. It is only by knowing precisely what our needs are that we can assure compliance in meeting those needs.

Staffing is the greatest challenge in our industry. We must set our standard high, determine what our staffing pattern should be and use every God-given ability to achieve and maintain that staffing pattern for our facility.

PEOPLE WILL STRIVE
TO LIVE UP TO
YOUR EXPECTATIONS OF
THEM

Chapter V

Selection, training and retention of personnel are among the most important duties of any supervisor in the nursing facility. Selection of personnel is very time-consuming with the review of applications, acquisition of references and the conducting of interviews. The selection process itself can be exasperating when turnover is frequent and a great amount of time is consumed in that process.

Retention of personnel is of utmost importance to the facility. Quality patient care is produced when associates are adequately oriented to the facility, apprised of their duties and responsibilities by means of formalized training programs, and taught the specific concept of quality assurance/continuous quality improvement. The goal is to teach each associate to consistently solve problems and develop new and better ways to produce quality patient care.

There are two distinctive indicators that must be actively monitored within the facility in order to improve retention of associates. These indicators are turnover and absenteeism. It is a valuable practice to keep a monthly list of associates who have resigned or who have been terminated, along with the reason for each occurrence. It is important to look for common factors relating to resignations and terminations and determine the necessary procedures that we, as managers, can employ to reduce that turnover in our facility. If information is tabulated on a monthly basis, we will be able to evaluate the progress of the facility from a factual perspective. I, personally, have had the opportunity to see a tremendous improvement in the retention of associates by utilizing this simple method of monitoring and creatively developing programs that produce results.

The turnover rate is determined by dividing the total number of associate resignations or terminations in a given month by the total number of associates in the nursing department. Graphing the given turnover rate on a monthly basis will provide a visual picture of what is taking place in the facility.

An example of a graph representing turnover follows.

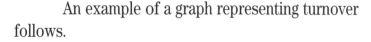

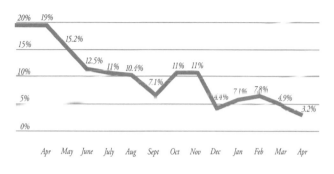

Turnover Rate

Let's remember that the healthiest competition is with ourselves. We must monitor the turnover rate in our facility, determine why nursing personnel is leaving and, most important, why they are staying. We must capitalize on their reasons for staying and resolve any common factors influencing their leaving. Believing that there is a way to resolve this issue, let's set about to find that way.

Absenteeism can be monitored and decreased in a similar fashion by making a list of all associates who have been absent during a given month and the number of absences for each one. By graphing absenteeism we can determine whether or not there is a distinct pattern of absenteeism for a particular associate and begin counseling him/her appropriately. We can calculate the percentage of absenteeism monthly by dividing the total number of shifts missed during that month by the total number of shifts scheduled during a given month and graph that percentage to obtain a visual picture of that concern in our facility.

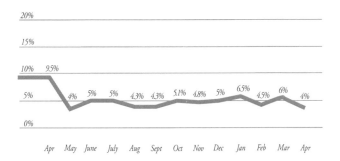

Absenteeism Rate

The Winner's Circle
The Circle of Love

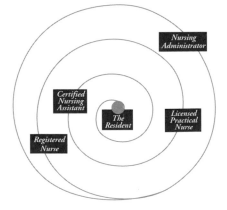

The Circle of Love must be unbroken
and never ending.

Associate morale is directly related to patient care. In order for patient care to be provided at its optimum level, and associate morale to be maintained at that same level, the mission, purpose and priority of the facility must be presented understandably to all associates. That mission, purpose and priority must be one that each associate can relate to and easily become a part of. The preceding circle pictures a way of presenting our philosophy to the associates. No matter how we present an organizational chart to our associates, someone always appears to be at the top and another one at the bottom. This automatically sets the stage for feelings of inferiority on the part of some associates. When this particular organizational structure is presented to the associates, it portrays a team approach—the ultimate goal of each part of the circle being the creation of an atmosphere of quality patient care.

The large Winner's Circle is made up of several smaller circles, each circle building upon the strength of the other connecting circle. Every circle is necessary for the wellbeing of the whole. The continuum and continuity of quality patient care as each nursing associate strives to perform his/her skill and job duties to his/her maximum potential. Each associate has a specific job duty to perform in order to keep the circle unbroken and constantly providing quality care. The circle remains intact and strong with low turnover, little absenteeism and a high level of education for each associate. With the implementation of this "circle of love," the patient is the ultimate winner.

When associates were asked what it would take to maintain that circle, the following comments were made: (a) An individual must have the desire, and be committed, to caring for the patients. (b) The associate must enjoy his/her work—job satisfaction is important. (c) You must have good rapport with co-workers. (d) The attitude of personnel must be positive—mistakes must be allowed. (e) We are like a family—we must work out our problems, not just complain. (f) Associates must not come to work angry or go home angry. (g) Job knowledge is very important. (h) Associates must love patients, be forbearing and have compassion for others.

It is imperative to monitor turnover and absenteeism rates monthly in order to identify problem areas, assess, clarify solutions and implement, thus decreasing these problems and producing a stronger circle and better patient care. Retention of associates is of utmost importance. The value of an associate who has been oriented and trained in the facility, who is familiar with all of the wants, needs, desires and idiosyncrasies of the residents is immeasurable. It takes months to re-establish the confidence that a resident has placed in an associate. That trust and confidence come only after months of day-to-day interaction. We may never be able to pay our associates what they are worth, but we can educate them to feel comfortable with their duties and responsibilities, give them an incentive to reach for a star, train them to view a problem as an opportunity to develop a unique solution, and discipline them as the term is meant to be applied—"to teach." As we help each of them grow and become the best person he or she can be, the entire facility will likewise grow and improve so as to produce the highest quality of care within reach of available resources.

We are confronted with two questions as we deal with the staffing issue in our facility. (1) What can I do within the walls of my facility to attain and maintain adequate staffing? (2) What impact will the procedures and management techniques that I employ have on other facilities in my area? As we philosophically discover ways to improve ourselves while being careful not to harm anyone else, we will resolve many issues and become the best that we can be.

SECTION II

PATIENT CARE

CHAPTER VI

NUTRITION AND THE ELDERLY

One area of concern when caring for the elderly is that of nutrition. How do we evaluate the nutritional status of our residents? What measures can we take to provide adequate nutrition for those who are under our care?

One obvious method of monitoring the nutritional status of a resident is by monitoring his/her weight. The question arises, "How can we best accomplish this task?" We learn very rapidly that to obtain an accurate weight evaluation is no simple task; it is an art and a science. In my experience, the best case scenario is to have one person trained in the art of weight monitoring. The ability to correctly balance the scales, to accurately subtract the weight of the wheelchair and several other technical skills must be carefully taught.

First and foremost, we must record a weight for each resident in our facility. The next step is to determine the ideal body weight for that resident. It is recommended that we compile a list of all residents consisting of their names, their ideal body weights and a spread sheet beginning in January and continuing through December. This information can assist us at a glance in identifying trends of specific variations in weight. The criteria for monitoring weight loss are:

1. List those residents who are 10 percent under ideal body weight.
2. List those residents who have had a five percent weight loss in the last 30 days.
3. List those residents who have lost 7.5 percent in the last 90 days.
4. List those residents who have had a 10 percent weight loss in the last 180 days.

As we monitor this criteria on a monthly basis, we can begin to feel knowledgeable about what is happening with our residents.

As residents are identified in these categories, it is recommended that we obtain weekly weights on them. Other things that can be discussed are lab data, three-day calorie counts, supplemental feedings, appetite stimulants, double portions, etc., as we look at ways to improve their nutritional status. It is important to keep staff apprised of the information gained by this monitoring. Small group meetings with licensed personnel and nursing assistants on a given wing will afford the opportunity to share information with our staff and in turn obtain information from them that could be beneficial in this endeavor.

In my experience, a system that produced quite positive results was to serve all of the residents in this category with a red tray. This is a simple approach to assist staff members in the identification of residents about whom we are concerned. It is suggested that we share this information with family members so that they are assured of our continued monitoring of weight loss in order to make certain their loved one is receiving adequate nutrition.

It is recommended that the director of nursing and the dietary supervisor meet on a weekly basis to discuss any concerns regarding the nutritional status of the residents. It is also recommended that the registered dietitian evaluate these residents on a monthly basis. Many times our elderly and/or their families become critical of the food in our facilities. This is understandable for various reasons, but we can assure them that we are providing adequate nutrition in every way possible.

A weighted question that comes to our mind, decidedly a quality of life issue, is, "Should our residents be placed on a therapeutic diet?" In November of 1989, all residents of the facility under my supervision as director of nursing were placed on a "Regular Diet, Texture as Tolerated." Within the facility we had 22 diabetics who were on special diets previous to this date. Twenty-five residents were previously on a low sodium diet and were diagnosed with congestive heart failure and/or hypertension. Two residents were on a bland diet for gastrointestinal disturbances. The criteria for evaluating these residents were:

1. Lab work three months previous to change
2. Lab work one week after residents were placed on diet
3. Lab work one month after residents were placed on diet
4. Record of symptoms one month previous to change
5. Record of symptoms one month after diet change

The results were:

DIABETICS

Two diabetics exhibited an increase in blood sugar that was above the normal range after the diets were started. Ninety percent exhibited a fasting blood sugar within a normal range one month after the implementation of the regular diets.

Congestive Heart Failure/Hypertension

Two residents exhibited an elevated blood pressure one month after the regular diets were implemented. One resident exhibited the symptom of increased edema after one month. Eighty-eight percent of the residents exhibited no change in blood pressure or any symptom related to their diet change.

Gastrointestinal Disturbances

Those residents who were on a bland diet previous to the implementation of the new diets exhibited no symptom or adverse reaction.

Another area of concern relating to the nutrition of our residents is the question regarding enteral feeding. This question must be answered for each of our residents on an individual basis from an ethical position. A very important part of that process is the documentation of how the decision is made for each resident.

GOOD, BETTER, BEST
NEVER LET IT REST
UNTIL
THE GOOD IS BETTER
AND
THE BETTER BEST

IF WE DO OUR BEST,
GOD WILL DO THE REST

Chapter VII

Hydration of the Elderly

A chronic concern about elderly people is the possibility of dehydration. Each resident placed under our care should receive a minimum of 1500 cc's of fluid over a 24-hour period of time. More specifically, the way to determine the actual fluid intake by each resident is by means of the following formula: Body weight in pounds divided by 2.2 multiplied by 30 equals total number of cc's of fluid required for a 24-hour period of time. The first thing we must decide is which of our residents has the potential for dehydration. It is recommended that the following specific categories of residents be monitored very closely for possible dehydration.

1. Residents requiring tube feedings
2. Residents having foley catheters
3. Residents who are underweight

4. Residents who are unable to obtain their own fluids
5. Residents receiving diuretic medications

Once we have decided which residents fall into these categories, the question arises, "How do we monitor these residents to determine if they are receiving an adequate amount of intake?" The first step in the process is to place them on intake and output. We must begin by measuring the amount of fluid intake for each individual resident (i.e. 1500 cc's of fluid per 24-hour period or an individually determined amount). If the resident has not been receiving an adequate amount of fluid intake, we need to encourage additional fluid intake and continue to monitor. If a resident continues for two consecutive days to lack adequate intake, we need to monitor for signs and symptoms of dehydration (poor skin turgor, dry mucous membranes, lab values such as specific gravity and BUNs) and report this to the physician. As we continue the process of monitoring and encouraging fluids, the number of residents diagnosed as dehydrated should decrease, although initially the number will probably increase. By monitoring our residents in this way on a continuous basis, we will begin to feel much more in control of this chronic problem.

The next question that comes to mind as we build this program is, "Who is responsible for completing the required tasks in order to cause this program to be totally implemented?" It would seem that our nursing assistants would be responsible for monitoring the actual intake and output. This should be documented on the resident's record by the charge nurse each shift. At the end of each 24-hour period, possibly each morning at 7:00 a.m., someone needs to be assigned the specific responsibility of totaling the 24-hour intake and output. This person may be either a trained nursing assistant, a ward clerk or a charge nurse. These totals should be reviewed each day by the charge nurse and/or the supervisor and recommendations made as required. Many facilities have recognized the need for a "hydration aide" position to assist in making sure that each resident is receiving an adequate fluid intake. When this system of monitoring dehydration is in place, the daily crisis of dealing with the acutely dehydrated resident should become a thing of the past. The residents will be receiving quality care and the nursing management will be more organized and efficient.

Chapter VIII

Rehabilitation of the Elderly

The frail elderly placed under our care need so little, but they need that little so much. So many of the functions we do everyday and take for granted no longer come so easy for them. This brings to our discussion the activities of daily living of our residents, better known as ADLs. This list of activities consists of bathing, dressing, eating, toileting and ambulation. How many of our residents can perform these activities on their own? How can we assist them in attaining as much independence as possible?

The accomplishment of this task requires a lot of education for our nursing staff. It is more important to encourage and assist our residents in doing it themselves than to do it for them. Each resident should be evaluated as to his/her individual ability to perform ADLs and then determine how assistance can be given in that performance so as to maximize the individual's level of independence.

Bathing our residents is an important part of their routine and quite a challenge for each of us to meet. I remember the first time I was confronted with that challenge. I began to appraise our situation: (a) How many of our residents need help with bathing? (b) How many baths should they have in a given week? (c) Who should be entrusted with the giving of those baths? (d) What kind of baths should they be given? (e) How can we document the fact that the baths have been given?

As we give attention to these questions, we can begin to individualize the specific bathing needs of each resident. If they can wash their own faces, let them do so. If a male resident can shave himself, let him perform that task. If a female resident is able to brush her hair, encourage her to do so. If we allow and encourage a resident to do for oneself when able, we help him or her feel more independent and thus improve each one's quality of life.

As we consider the subject of dressing our residents, again we ask, what can they accomplish by themselves? The response to this question can include everything from completely dressing themselves to helping choose the clothes they wish to wear for the day.

Mealtime and eating become the highlight of our resident's day. Many times this event is the one function at which a resident can maintain some autonomy for a longer period of time. Again we question their abilities from the act of feeding themselves without assistance to the opposite extreme of being totally tube fed without any involvement of their own. If we are prone to question the importance of allowing a resident to feed him/her self with any kind of device available, then we need to permit someone to feed us an entire meal. This experience will not only help us understand the importance of allowing the resident to maintain his/her independence in eating, but will also give insight regarding the best way to feed a resident if it becomes necessary.

Is the resident continent or incontinent with reference to the bowel and/or bladder? Does he/she suffer from chronic constipation and/or impactions? Are we doing everything possible to assist our residents in maintaining as much independence as possible in the area of toileting? Have we assessed each resident's need for bowel and bladder training? Does the staff understand all that is involved in a bowel and bladder training program? One factor to consider is the importance of establishing a pattern for residents, not a routine for staff, as we attempt a retraining program. If a resident cannot be retrained, we can establish a staff routine to keep him/her as clean and dry as possible. A program that can be implemented along this line is a bowel management program. This can be quite successful in the prevention of constipation and/or impaction for those residents who are prone to have either of these conditions. This program consists mainly of the use of fiber in the diet, the encouragement of taking in fluids during the day, the increase in exercise whenever possible, the provision of stool softeners on a daily basis, and the administering of suppositories at least three days a week.

The inability to ambulate can be a real concern of our residents. It is not only an issue of independence, but also a potential problem of the occurrence of complications such as skin breakdown, contractures or the decrease in the functioning ability systems because of the lack of mobility. What measures can be taken to ensure independence and self ambulation whenever possible? If the resident demands total care and is in need of specific positioning, can he/she transfer from bed to chair or ambulate with the assistance of a walker, cane, etc.?

As we consider the activities of daily living for our residents and their individual needs, it is not only valuable to address each resident on an individual basis, but also to examine their needs collectively to determine staffing needs for quality care and the educational programs necessary to equip our staff for the tasks they must perform.

Elderly residents have the very same needs that each of us has. It becomes our responsibility to provide the programs to meet those needs on a daily basis, thus ensuring a quality of life for each of them.

As we staff our facilities with a full-time staff of physical, speech, and occupational therapists, we will certainly be better positioned to provide a quality of life to our residents.

CHAPTER IX

PHYSICAL RESTRAINT REDUCTION

PHYSICAL RESTRAINT: Effective January 1990, the Federal Register (SS483.23) states: "Physical restraints <u>are</u> any manual method or physical or mechanical device, material or equipment attached or adjacent to the resident's body that the individual cannot remove easily which restricts freedom of movement or normal access to one's body."

OUR PHILOSOPHY: The least restrictive product is always the best product possible. The more freedom the patient has, the better it is for his/her health and psychological well-being. Only when the patient is in danger of injury to him/her self or others is the restraint applicable.

RATIONALE: The Omnibus Budget Reconciliation Act of 1987 (OBRA) specifies that "the resident has the right to be free from any physical restraints imposed, or psychoactive drug administered for purposes of discipline or convenience, and not required to treat the resident's medical symptoms." It further states, "Restraints may only be imposed to ensure the physical safety of the resident or other residents, and only upon the written order of a physician that specifies the duration and circumstances under which the restraints are to be used (except in emergency situations that must be addressed in the facility's restraint)." Therefore, nursing home staff must be more discriminant in the use of both chemical and physical restraints, reducing or eliminating their use whenever possible.

Previous to the OBRA regulations, it was not uncommon to see 40 percent to 60 percent of our residents physically restrained in our facilities. At this point in time, the average percentage of physical restraints is more like 15 percent. Facilities across the country have reached zero percent physical restraint utilization.

Zofia Long, a regional vice president for Life Care Centers of America in the New England regions, has guided her entire region to zero percent physical restraint utilization.

Detrimental Effects of Physical (PR) and Chemical (CR) Restraints on Residents developed by the National Citizens' Coalition for Nursing Home Reform for the National Center for State Long-Term Care Ombudsman Resources funded by the Administration on Aging

EFFECT	CAUSE	PREVENTION
Skin Bruising/cuts/redness (PR)	Incorrectly applied restraint or improper size or type of restraint. Resident struggles against restraint.	Apply restraint correctly according to manufacturer's direction. Use alternative methods. Apply restraint for short periods only. Release, exercise, at least every two hours—more often if necessary. Use alternative methods.
Pressure ulcers (PR/CR)	Resident in one position too long. Studies show two times number of pressure ulcers in restrained residents.	

PSYCHOLOGICAL

Panic/anxious expression/combative/ increased confusion (PR/CR)	Frightened by PR. Does not like restraints. Does not understand why they are being used. Paradoxical reaction to a psychoactive drug; that is, it has the opposite effect intended. Person gives up when restrained, withdraws, broken spirit, staff ignores restrained resident. Drug in too large dose.	Use alternative methods. Use CR and PR for short periods only. Use different drug, lower dose or no drug.
Lethargy/depression/ decreased social interaction (PR/CR)		Use alternative methods. Increase opportunity to socialize. Frequent staff interaction. Decrease time the restraint is used. Decrease drug dose or change drug.
Screaming/yelling/calling out (CR/PR)		Use alternative options, identify and meet needs, comfort.

GASTRO INTESTINAL
GENITO-URINARY

Decrease in appetite/weight loss/sunken cheek bones/sores around mouth (CR/PR)	Broken spirit/not interested in life. Discomfort of restraint/preoccupation with discomfort. No activity to work up appetite. Too drowsy from drug use to eat.	Use alternative methods. Release, exercise at least every two hours. Decrease drug dose.
Dehydration/dry skin/dry mouth/sunken eyes/fever/acute confusion. (CR/PR)	Cannot reach water. Too drowsy to drink. Too depressed to drink. Does not recognize decreased sense of thirst.	Use alternative methods. Leave water within reach at all times. Offer fluids/encourage to drink between meals and at mealtime.

Urinary tract infections (CR/PR). Pain and frequency of urination, fever.	Catheter use, not regularly, low fluid intake.	Toilet to avoid incontinence, increase fluid intake, use alternative methods.
Constipation/impaction. Resident complains of stomach ache/constipation restlessness. Decreased appetite/confusion/pre-occupied with bowels. (CR/PR)	Lack of activity. Inability to get enough fluids. Not taken to bathroom according to lifelong bowel pattern.	Release, exercise, toilet every two hours or more often if necessary. Toilet according to lifelong pattern. Offer fluids between and at meals. Leave water within reach. Use alternative methods.

RESPIRATORY

Resident complains that chest feels tight/says he can't breathe/appears anxious.	Chest/vest restraint is too tight. Resident fears restraint and has anxiety attack.	Use alternative methods. Loosen restraint. Decrease use of drugs. Exercise every two hours or more if necessary.
Pneumonia (CR/PR) Acute confusion/shortness of breath/chest pain.	Lack of movement allows secretions to pool, decreases efficiency of lungs with decreased oxygen exchange and increased confusion. Shortness of breath when active.	Same as above.

PLAN

All residents having a physical restraint in place will be evaluated to determine the necessity of the restraint.

PROCEDURE

1. Evaluation of each resident to determine the type of restraint utilized and the reason for that restraint.
2. Consultation with the resident's physician to receive the appropriate order (may use alternatives of the facility's choice regarding the restraint).
3. The original order will be written by the nurse receiving the order.
4. The order will be brought forward each month on the newly printed physician's orders.
5. All members of the staff will be made aware of those residents who are involved in the restraint reduction program.
6. Residents will be continuously evaluated by nursing and therapy to insure that the least necessary restrictive restraint device is used.

DEFINITIONS

Restraint/restrictive products: Those products that limit or deter the range of motion or the freedom to act on the part of the patient. Most safety products and postural supports may be considered restrictive. Conversely, if a patient is able to apply or release a safety device, it would not be considered a restraint.

MEDICAL AUTHORITY

The Medical Authority is a combination of a medical doctor's opinion with the consideration of pertinent facts provided by the facility's executive director, nursing staff and family. Opinion is transferred into action when a doctor writes an order or a prescription for a specific device and designates its use.

CHAPTER X

RESPIRATORY THERAPY

When we become a director of nursing in long-term care, we are a bit unnerved when faced with the responsibilities of this area. I remember my reaction when I first realized I was responsible for the delivery of oxygen to my residents. While working in a hospital, it was a simple matter to pick up the phone and call respiratory therapy when I needed them. I remember thinking, what is an oxygen concentrator and where do I obtain one? How many do I need for this facility? I do remember something about being sure that 02 cylinders are firmly secured so they can't fall over, and–oh, yes– we do need signs that don't allow smoking when oxygen is in use.

We learn that it is important to be knowledgeable about which residents are receiving oxygen. It is recommended to make a list of residents charting the following questions:

(a) Is the resident receiving 02 PRN or continuous? (b) How are we documenting the utilization of 02 in the facility? (c) What is the procedure required by infection control policy to make certain the residents are not becoming infected from the use of 02? (d) How do we protect our residents from skin breakdown that may occur from the use of 02 tubing? As we ponder these thoughts and formulate answers, we develop a workable program for the basics of respiratory therapy in our facility.

As we progress toward the development of in-house respiratory therapy programs, our residents will be better served and we will be able to provide care for the resident who requires a more aggressive respiratory therapy program.

CHAPTER XI

PRESSURE ULCER PREVENTION

In reviewing the anatomy of the skin, we learn that the skin is the largest organ of the body. The skin receives one-third of the total blood supply of the body. The two layers of the skin are known as the epidermis, the nonvascular outer layer of the skin, and the dermis, the second layer of the true skin. Beneath the epidermis is found the subcutaneous tissue, muscle and bone.

A dermal ulcer is defined as an area of the skin where the lack of blood flow has caused an area of cellular nercrosi (death). A dermal ulcer may be classified as a pressure ulcer. A pressure ulcer is defined as an area of skin where pressure has progressively destroyed the soft tissue.

There are four stages described according to pathological involvement:

Stage I	Inflammation or reddening of the skin.
Stage II	Skin blister or superficial skin break.
Stage III	Full thickness skin loss exposing subcutaneous tissue.
Stage IV	Full thickness skin loss exposing muscle or bone.

The characteristics of pressure ulcers are:

1. **Inflammation**
   Reaction of tissue to injury. Classical signs are pain, heat, redness and swelling.
2. **Undermining**
   To necrose supporting materials from under the skin.
3. **Eschar**
   A thick, leathery, black crust of dead tissue, often covering an underlying necrotic process.
4. **Slough**
   Strong-like necrotic debris that may be yellow, grey or green in color.

The documentation regarding pressure ulcers should always include the following information: stage, location, size, appearance, drainage, odor, inflammation and undermining. The systematic approach to management of pressure ulcers consists of:

1. Understanding the problem
2. Preplanning
3. Consistency and continuity
4. Planning of care to include (a) assessment, (b) intervention and (c) evaluation.

Basic considerations for treatment of pressure ulcers are:

STANDARD

Facility personnel will administer appropriate care and treatment in order to heal existing pressure ulcers and prevent the development of new pressure ulcers.

GOAL

100 percent of all post admission pressure ulcers will be noted and healed at Stage I.

POLICY

(Name of facility) shall evaluate all residents upon admission and on an ongoing basis in order to identify those who have pressure ulcers and/or have potential for pressure ulcers. Prevention protocol as well as treatment protocol shall be established and followed. Staff shall be sufficiently trained in order to identify, treat and prevent occurrence of pressure ulcers. Monitoring of all residents having pressure ulcers and/or potential for pressure ulcers shall be completed on a weekly basis to determine the status of those residents at that point in time. Treatment regimens and prevention protocol will be evaluated as to their success and revised as necessary. The status of all pressure ulcers shall be reported monthly to the Quality Assurance Committee and the overall program shall be evaluated to ensure a continuous, progressive and successful program.

PROCEDURE

1. Identify all residents who have potential for skin breakdown.
2. Determine the necessary protocol for implementing a program for the prevention of pressure ulcers.
   (a) Whirlpool bath daily at the first sign of a reddened area.
3. Determine the protocol for the treatment of pressure ulcers.

CHAPTER XII

ALZHEIMER'S DISEASE
November 14, 1986

I walked into the hallway and there he stood,
surrounded by nursing personnel. He was frightened,
combative and wanting to leave. The tension
surrounding him was enormous. I walked up to his
side and stood there quietly listening to him speak of
leaving, of no one touching him and, in general,
words that denoted fear. I knew from what he was
saying that he was afraid—afraid of walls and the
people around him that were unfamiliar to him. I
knew his feelings were in control of him now and
there was no way of logically communicating with
him at this point. After allowing him the opportunity
to air his emotions for a period of time, without
restraint, I simply walked along beside him, noting
that as I physically obstructed a particular path, he
would turn in another direction. At one point, I
placed my hand very gently on his arm, being

careful to convey feelings of calm reassurance, genuine concern and compassion in my touch. We walked along the hallway and I very gently led him to a chair at the end of the hallway. With a light touch on his arm, I suggested that he sit down. Once he was seated in the chair, I sat down on the floor in front of him. With my hand on his, I looked into his eyes to convey reassurance and compassion. He continued to talk and, at times, would grit his teeth to show anger. I steadfastly guarded my feelings and, holding his hand, looked into his eyes, relaying the message, "It's okay and I care about you." I really do not know the time span of this entire occurrence, but eventually, without speaking a word, I was able, only by utilizing the senses of touch and sight and the transference of feelings, to dissolve his anger. The calmness, concern and compassion prevailed and he went peacefully to sleep.

Alzheimer's disease is a progressive, irreversible, neurological disorder that affects an estimated 2.5 million American adults. It is the most common form of dementing illness. Alzheimer's disease causes 150,000 deaths annually and is the fourth leading cause of death in adults, after heart disease, cancer and stroke.

Over the past few years we have increased our knowledge of the symptoms, diagnosis, staging and management of this disease. We have learned that there is "life after the diagnosis of Alzheimer's disease." If we utilize certain management concepts that are unique to the demented patient, his/her quality of life can be improved.

We are aware of the rapid acceleration of the elderly population and the increase in Alzheimer's disease. We have reviewed studies that demonstrate the improvement in the quality of life that can be achieved in a specialized Alzheimer's disease unit. Symptoms of the disease are as follows: (a) apraxia, (b) wandering, (c) catastrophic reaction, (d) disorientation, (e) forgetfulness, (f) seizures, (g) withdrawal, (h) hallucination/delusion, (i) anomia, (j) apathy and depression, (k) suspicion and paranoia, (l) agnosia, (m) inappropriate sexual behavior and (n) perseveration.

The concept of an "emotionally controlled environment" will allow the patient to wander freely without the threat of physical and chemical restraints and will allow the patient the freedom to make mistakes, have a catastrophic reaction, whatever he or she feels like doing, and will still be loved, respected and cared for by the staff.

We must learn to deal with their feelings. The Alzheimer's disease patient can no longer cope with situations by understanding logic or reasoning. We can control certain situations only by understanding their feelings. The goal for an Alzheimer's unit is to provide an environment conducive to the management and treatment of the Alzheimer's disease patient. The objectives of the Alzheimer's disease unit are:

1. To provide an environment free from chemical or physical restraint for the patient whose diagnosis is Alzheimer's disease.
2. To provide a support group for family members and/or significant other persons who assist in caring for the Alzheimer's disease patient.
3. To provide appropriate training for staff members in the management and treatment of the Alzheimer's patient. This includes the initial classroom instruction and an ongoing in-service program.
4. To develop plans to control difficult behavior resulting from the illness.

The caregiver is faced with the problem of (a) understanding as much as possible about the disease itself, and (b) dealing with the constant demands of the emotional environment. The caregiver must become a "saint," having constant control of his/her own feelings and behavior.

We need to be understanding of the family members, not judgmental or condemning. Awareness of what they have been dealing with day after day before bringing their loved one to the facility is a must. It is humanly impossible to physically care for and emotionally care about a person who has so many demands 24 hours a day, seven days a week, 52 weeks a year. It is our job to provide that ray of hope in what appears to be a hopeless situation. We can do this by becoming a resource person who can help the family member find some specific answers for many questions and by our presence assure him or her that we understand that it is okay. The family is as much our responsibility as is the patient. We must try to deal with their problems and provide a better quality of life for all concerned. The code of ethics we strive to maintain in caring for the elderly is: (a) We do nothing for the patient that he/she is able to do for him/her self. It is our responsibility to insist that the resident perform all of those ADLs he or she is capable of performing in order to keep the senses as keen as possible, and to keep muscles from becoming atrophic. (b) We will help the elderly by treating, managing or preventing problems that could adversely affect quality of life in old age. The loss of the ability to control body functions, the loss of memory and the loss of agility are prominent examples of the problem. (c) We will supplement the care given by relatives and try to prevent a breakdown of those informal support systems. (d) We will help the elderly have a peaceful death as well as a good life.

Patient abuse is not just a horror story we hear about through the media. It is sometimes insidious and, unfortunately, we may be guilty of such abuse without realizing it. Our interpretation of patient abuse is perhaps a bit more stringent than the regulations. If we view the residents as precious individuals with individual wants and needs, treating them as we would our own mom or dad, we should not have a problem in any of these areas.

The process of aging is a normal course of life. Our society in general tends to "closet" the elderly. This is characterized by the TV commercials we see. The old people we see are not "old;" they aren't wrinkled, crippled, paralyzed, incontinent or depressed. Those people are affluent, bright and their greatest medical problem is, "Which laxative should I buy?" We see the "real" world of aging everyday. We see the fear, the uncertainty and the depression. Our goal is to remove the sadness from their eyes by showing compassion and respect. We learn from them by listening and observing their silent communication. As we work with the elderly, we must give them a sense of belonging, because in some cases, we are all they have left. They must be given the right of self-determination and we are responsible for activating their motivation to reach those self-determined goals.

Several steps in this process are as follows:
1. Help them set their goals.
2. Assist them in reaching those goals.
3. Assist them in maintaining their dignity and personal identity.
4. Through loving care, teach them to continue to love in return.

The severely demented are faced with the physical problems of eating, dressing, sleeping, bathing, going to the bathroom, apraxia, wandering and catastrophic reactions, to mention a few. Many of these simple daily routines that we take for granted are very complicated, frustrating, almost insurmountable tasks for these individuals. Our job is to observe, identify and assist the resident in accomplishing these tasks.

The seven stages of cognitive decline are identified as:

Level I	Normal	No subjective or objective changes in intellectual functioning with increasing age.
Level II	Normal Aged	Subjective discomfort, forgetfulness, no overt emotional symptoms (prognosis is benign).

Level III	Early Confusion	Begins to interfere at work and in social situations. Memory loss at this stage frequently is accompanied by a marked increase in anxiety.
Level IV	Late Confusion	Early Alzheimer's disease. Person loses the ability to handle such routine activities as marketing or managing personal and household finances. Denial is the dominant defense mechanism and the patient withdraws emotionally.
Level V	Early Dementia	Can no longer survive alone in the community. Most of the time, denial mercifully protects the patient from confronting the terrible truth that he is literally "losing his mind." Still on occasion anger, suspicion and transient crying episodes occur.

Level VI	Middle Dementia	Begins to require assistance with such basic activities of daily life as bathing and toileting. The world becomes frightening to patients at this stage, and the chemical balance in the brain changes markedly. For these psychological and neurochemical reasons, denial becomes less effective. Instead of withdrawal, the patient is prone to agitation, violence, paranoia and delusions. For example, he may talk to imaginary people or accuse the spouse of being an impostor. Emotional changes in this stage are variable and can also include obsessive symptoms, such as repeating a cleaning activity. The patient shows a loss in willpower because he cannot carry a thought long enough to determine an action.

Level VII	Late Dementia	First loses the ability to speak and then to walk. The end stages are stupor and coma. In most cases, denial again protects patients against much of the emotional impact of the illness. In some patients, denial is so effective in the late dementia phase that the patient may continue to laugh, smile and appear to enjoy life as much as anyone else. The victim even at the late stage is often as kindly and amenable, as recalcitrant and angry as he/she ever was.

It has been brought to our attention that the needs of the Alzheimer's disease patients are very different from those of the "normal" population of patients in the nursing home environment. We understand that these patients are very special and have very unique needs and, therefore, we have developed management concepts that can meet these needs. We are reminded that we are the ones with the good mind that can change and adapt, and it is important that we know the rules and be creative in following them. A successful Alzheimer's disease unit will be achieved only by the flexibility of the staff. A part of learning to cope in nursing is learning to accept the fact that many patients will never recover, despite anything we can do. Alzheimer's disease is entirely and hopelessly debilitating. The reward in caring for such a patient comes from knowing that we have helped the resident hold onto his world as long as possible. In our relationships with people on the job, it is imperative that we work together to maintain an environment conducive to the care and treatment of the Alzheimer's disease patient. If we "do what we value and value what we do," we will feel good about ourselves and then be able to enhance the feelings of others.

The valuing steps are as follows:
1. **Choosing–**
   From alternatives
   Freely
   After careful consideration of the
   consequences
2. **Prizing–**
   Being proud of or glad about our choice
   Being willing to share or disclose our
   choice to others
3. **Acting–**
   Choices are reflected in behavior
   On the choice that is exhibited repeatedly
   and consistently

The test of our learning and understanding about Alzheimer's disease will begin when the first patient walks through the door, and it will continue day after day as we implement our concepts, monitor and adjust to meet the needs of our patients. We must remember that this is a totally new concept, and we are the pioneers in the management of Alzheimer's disease. We must be willing to constantly evaluate what we are doing and decide if we are giving the best possible care that could be provided for these special people. The real test lies in what happens to these patients once they are placed within our care.

LET'S REMEMBER–

Life is full of problems. Sometimes they are small ones that try our patience, and sometimes larger ones that try our souls.

We learn that we can be rendered weak and helpless, searching for the real meaning of life. To have special friends and loved ones nearby becomes an obsession. We fear being alone.

To realize that the only reason we can find for our own survival is the fact that someone cares for us, loves and needs us.

To ask our creator "Why?" but receive no answer except "be patient, have faith and the answer will come."

To learn to take life one day, one hour, one moment at a time because that may be all that we have. To be afraid that your heart will become cold and hard because of the hurt and pain within your body.

To say and do things we don't really mean and later pray for forgiveness.

To know the feeling of real depression and guilt.

To finally decide that the only thing which matters in life is to love—to love those who care for us, love those who love us, love our enemies and, most of all, to love ourselves because that is the way God meant it to be—knowing that we are created in

His image. If we can come through all of our problems, large or small, and still be loving, caring and giving, we have truly succeeded in overcoming the obstacles in our path.

We must never stop loving, because that's what it is all about.

CHAPTER XIII

DRUG UTILIZATION AND THE ELDERLY

When an elderly lady was admitted to the long-term care facility, she was taking 17 different medications. She was prone to fits of rage and screaming and even suffered episodes of delusion. Under the care of the staff at the facility, her medications were reduced to one, and she now uses her mouth for smiling instead of screaming.

This case is not unusual. Overmedication is a problem gaining more and more attention on both a state and federal level, and rightfully so. Each year, according to the American Hospital Association, 73,000 thousand elderly Americans die from drug overuse or misuse. That is more than the total number of American fatalities during the war in Vietnam.

My medical director, Dr. J.W. Colinger, and I were afforded a great opportunity. The two of us were privileged to appear before the United States Senate Special Committee on Aging to discuss the problems of drug overuse and to present the program we had instituted in our facility to cut down the number of medications utilized by the residents. "Basically, our philosophy was that we would not give any patient any kind of drug that was not absolutely needed." We saw a very successful rate of drug reduction through the exercise of that philosophy. A significant educational process of making the staff and families familiar with our goals was instituted. The facility kept the average number of medications per patient in a range from 3.1 to 3.7 for over a year. These figures were well below the national average of 6.1.

Additionally, through specialized management in the Alzheimer's disease unit, the staff was able to successfully decrease or eliminate 86 percent of the antipsychotic medications used in that area of the facility.

The federal committee learned of the facility's low drug usage from a report filed by the facility with the Medicaid Medical Advisory Board in Nashville. The rationale for the development of the program and the results of it, which were fairly dramatic in relationship to relieving people of unnecessary medications, was explained to the Senate Committee. Although the emphasis of the committee's probe was aimed at drug overuse and drug interactions, the committee was also concerned with the information available to doctors concerning drug implications among the elderly. The committee has had a long, running battle with the Food and Drug Administration regarding labeling in the PDR (Physician's Desk Reference) for geriatric indications. It also wanted drug companies to put geriatric dosing and prescribing information as a separate category, as they do for pediatrics

Because older adults generally have more health problems, drug overuse is a bigger problem for them. The older adult's body is biologically different from its youthful status. The capacity to eliminate drugs from the body is reduced with age, thus the propensity to have problems is increased.

Problems of drug overuse stem from a number of factors. Elderly patients often have many doctors, and the patients do not always tell their doctors about the prescriptions they are already taking. This can lead to duplication of drugs and drug interaction problems. Lack of patient education, over-prescribing by some doctors and drug-seeking behavior by certain patients are also factors in the overuse of drugs.

Since the implementation of the drug program, several of the patients that became bedridden are now ambulatory. They are happier, they eat better and their quality of life has been improved markedly. In addition to the improved quality of life for the patients, this program could also effect a financial savings. We calculated a savings to Medicare/Medicaid of over $15 million a year if all nursing homes in Tennessee could reduce from 7 to 3.2 the average number of drugs per patient.

Drug utilization review should be an integral aspect of quality assurance in all nursing home facilities. This review process should utilize a multidisciplinary approach that involves the medical director, director of nursing, executive director and other allied personnel. We accomplished this review by using a four-step process beginning with the arrival of the patient at our facility and continuing concurrently through his/her discharge. The steps are:

> 1. Development of the patient's problem list. An accurate determination of each patient's diagnoses and problems upon admission is a critical starting point in the overall management of the nursing home patient. This is accomplished by means of a careful review of the patient's medical records with a complete history and physical examination, and by obtaining appropriate laboratory tests.

2. Initial evaluation of drug utilization in relation to the problem list. Nursing home patients in particular and the elderly in general are clinically challenging to any physician. As people age, most disease processes are increasingly prevalent and the potential array of available medications is complex. Patients suffering from drug side effects and polypharmacy are all too common upon admission to a facility. After a problem list has been developed, a review of the patient's present medications is performed. If the patient is on unnecessary medications, these are discontinued.

3. Concurrent drug utilization review. Drug utilization at our facility is monitored using a two-step approach. Monthly, at the time of the physician-patient visit, medications are reviewed with the director of nursing and any deletions or additions are made. Additionally, at our monthly staff meeting, a facility-wide report was given to review the following: (a) duplication of medications—multiple medications being given for the same problem; i.e., a patient receiving two antidepressant medications; (b) PRN abuse—medications that are ordered on an as-needed basis and are

given routinely; (c) medications vs. diagnosis—the diagnosis does not justify a particular medication; (d) more than seven medications—any patient who is receiving more than seven regular medications has his/her chart reviewed by the medical director and, if necessary, is discussed with the attending physician; (e) narcotic medications—the charts of patients receiving this class medication are reviewed for appropriateness; (f) a facility-wide report is given for the average number of medications per patient and the previous month's comparison is noted; (g) a facility-wide report is given for the percentage of patients receiving antipsychotic medications and the previous month's comparison noted.

Through the use of this drug utilization program, our patients have been maintained on far less medication than the national average (6.1 vs. 3.1 to 3.7 per patient).

Intense research by the Institute for Health Systems Management indicates that there is a serious lack of adequate training about medication use with the elderly. The lack of education has resulted in ineffective treatment of patients, wasting of large amounts of money by health care facilities, and staggering health services over medication costs for the elderly. One area of specific concern is that of utilization of antipsychotic medications such as Haldol, Thorazine, Mellaril, etc. It is estimated that 60 percent of our elderly population of residents in nursing facilities are administered this type of medication for various reasons.

Residents receiving certain types of medication are placed at a higher risk for the development of possible side effects and adverse reactions. The adverse reactions and side effects of antipsychotic agents need to be reduced as much as possible in the nursing home environment. Adverse reactions such as extrapyramidal reactions— neuromuscular reactions have been reported frequently. In most residents, these reactions involved Parkinson-like symptoms that, when first observed, were usually mild to moderately severe and usually reversible. Other types of neuromuscular reactions (motor restlessness), dystonia, okathisia, hyperreflexia, opisthotonos, oculogyric crisis, (see attached list of definitions) have been reported far less frequently, but were often more severe.

All antipsychotic agents have been associated with persistent dyskinesias. Tardive dyskinesia may appear in some patients on long-term therapy. The risk appears to be greater in elderly patients on high-dose therapy, especially females. The symptoms are persistent and in some patients appear irreversible. There is no known effective treatment for tardive dyskinesia. Other central nervous system effects may include insomnia, restlessness, anxiety, euphoria, agitation, drowsiness, depression, lethargy, headache, confusion, vertigo, grandmal seizures, exacerbation of psychotic symptoms, including hallucinations and catatonic-like behavioral states, which may be responsive to drug withdrawal and/or treatment with anticholenergic drugs.

Quality of life becomes the issue. The utilization of antipsychotic medications can decrease the functional status of the elderly person to one who is unable to perform any of the daily duties that are required to survive in our world today. The resident who has the ability to walk, to feed himself, to bathe himself, etc., can become completely dependent upon those around him to meet these daily needs because of the administration of these medications; or, if you will, because of these "chemical restraints." A catastrophic reaction or a temporary agitation does not necessarily indicate long-term maintenance on antipsychotic medications.

The proposal to change, or decrease the utilization of these medications in a nursing facility, is: The facility is to institute a drug reduction program within the facility. The nursing staff must understand the purpose and importance of the drug reduction program and therefore have a positive attitude in regard to it. Many of the residents may have no change in behavior. A certain percentage may exhibit symptoms of agitation and be started again on the medications. In one month's period of time, those residents may again be evaluated. The initial evaluation establishes a baseline. One case history to note is that of an elderly female resident who was placed on the medication after several days of being agitated and several nights of insomnia. The resident was resting at night, but was continuing to be loud and agitated during the day with .05 mg's of Haldol twice a day. It would have appeared that increasing the dosage might have been helpful, but, instead, she became much quieter and much more alert when the Haldol was discontinued. The change program utilized in this plan is to increase the awareness, increase the knowledge of the importance of decreasing antipsychotic medications, and educate as to "how to" accomplish the task.

The overall philosophy of this program must be taught to and accepted by top management in the facility. This management team usually consists of the executive director, director of nursing and the physicians involved in the care of the residents. This organizational structure within itself causes some real concern in the process of change within the facility. Complications are added to the process because of the interaction of those concerned. The first step must be to educate the executive director, director of nursing, and the medical director of the facility.

It is felt that this would be accomplished most efficiently in a group meeting session, allowing input from each of these three entities, thus alleviating as much as possible the potential feeling of the need to defend one's turf. The quality of care and the quality of life of the resident must constantly remain the issue. The system by which this can be achieved in the most productive manner must be taught. Time is of a crucial nature in most facilities. A key indicator in this system is the fact that this can be accomplished systematically with very little increase in time on the part of top management. Once the philosophy and the systematic monitoring of the program is established within the facility, this goal can be achieved. The specific details of the program will be: (a) meet with top management, (b) meet with department heads within the facility, (c) meet with licensed nursing personnel, (d) meet with all nursing personnel, (e) inform residents and family members of the program, (f) establish the initial monitoring system, and (g) establish an ongoing monitoring system. The director of nursing and/or the medical director will be responsible for educating the attending physicians regarding the program.

THE ELDERLY NEED
SO LITTLE
BUT
THEY NEED THAT
LITTLE
SO VERY MUCH

SECTION III

QUALITY ASSURANCE

CHAPTER XIV

PROBLEM SOLVING

Problems are a part of life. As long as there are people, there will be problems. People are different in the manner in which they deal with problems. Some see a problem as a brick wall that they cannot get over, under, around or through. Others see a problem as a challenge they can meet, a difficulty that can become an opportunity. Each time that we as individuals learn to apply a problem-solving technique to a given situation in our lives, we discover more and more opportunities that are ours to enjoy. An important point to remember is that we can learn how to solve them and, each time we are able to solve a problem, we become more positive in our outlook and more powerful in our day-to-day living. Ten basic steps in problem solving are:

     1. Assume a logical, workable solution.

     2. Use only positive language.

3. Define the situation in writing.
4. List all possible causes of the situation.
5. List all possible solutions to the situation.
6. Make a clear, specific decision.
7. Assign specific responsibility for implementing the decision.
8. Set a deadline for implementing the necessary action.
9. Take action.
10. Follow up.

The first step in problem solving is to convince yourself that there is a logical, workable solution to the problem. If you do not believe that you and those around you have the ability and the motivation for solving any given problem in your environment, then your own attitude and mind-set is the problem. When a problem is shared with a group of people who collectively agree that they can solve a special problem, the positive force behind their mind-set will evolve into a solution and provide the energy to perform that solution.

The second stage of problem solving is to use only positive language in working toward a solution. This seems simple and elementary but if we carefully examine our speech, how much positive language do we actually use? I often wonder if we should take a course in the use of positive language as we would in French or German. If we learn to categorize a situation in such a way that it can give direction toward the solution, then we can speak more positively about the problem. For example, I believe that 99 percent of the people do not do things wrong on purpose, as I already stated in an earlier chapter. The reason things go wrong is because there is a lack of knowledge, a lack of skill, a lack of time management or a lack of priority. This approach puts the solution in our hands. These elements we can teach and bring the problem into focus. This philosophy produces results. The only time it cannot operate effectively is if the person does not "want to" solve the problem. That will take more thought and effort to bring about the desired result, but I believe this mind-set is the exception rather than the rule. Most people want to do a good job and receive recognition for it. A big part of our job as managers is to make sure that they have the opportunity to obtain the knowledge and training to perform successfully. We do not need to spend our valuable time "blaming and complaining." God has given us only so many hours in a day and a certain amount of energy. If we misuse that time and energy, we will not be able to make progress and move forward.

As we continue our discussion of the process of problem solving, the next step is to define the situation in writing. Many times when our emotions become involved in the problem, it becomes very beneficial to write it down and bring it into focus in our minds—thus relaxing the emotion. I think we will discover that it can help to develop a more objective viewpoint regarding the situation.

Listing all of the possible causes of a situation can assist us in determining which direction we should take in finding the solution. One note of caution at this point is we should not allow ourselves to include persons as possible causes. We are reminded, "If we point a finger at someone else, we point three fingers back at ourselves." After listing the causes of a problem, the list of all possible solutions be placed beside them. It is a good idea to "brainstorm" to develop creative ideas and measures for correcting the situation. Following that, we should evaluate and categorize all of these ideas so that we can determine the most plausible solutions.

We must make clear and positive decisions so that everyone involved will know exactly what is to be accomplished. Assigning specific responsibility helps everyone involved feel that they individually have a part in working out the solution. They will be fully knowledgeable about their responsibility and challenge in solving the problem.

Setting a deadline for implementing the solution gives everyone a goal to work toward and assures that the implementation process will begin and end as scheduled. The greatest solution in the world cannot produce results unless we take "action" to apply it. In following up, we need to monitor the situation to determine whether or not the best decisions have been made and the most effective measures have been taken to resolve the problem. Has the problem actually been solved for all persons involved? If not, what could we have done differently to bring about a better situation?

We have learned that problem-solving is an ongoing process. It is very valuable to train each associate in the problem-solving technique. If every associate is actively involved in problem-solving, we will be blessed with many more solutions and fewer problems. This will definitely be to our advantage.

We will not have perfection, although we continue to strive for it, but we can work together cooperatively toward our common goal.

LIFE IS FULL OF
PROBLEMS...
IN THE MIDDLE OF
DIFFICULTY
LIES OPPORTUNITY

CHAPTER XV

CONFLICT MANAGEMENT

Conflict is inevitable. Conflict is okay. It is normal for one human being to disagree with another in a given situation. In fact, many times conflict produces positive results. As we learn to manage conflict, we come to believe the proverb that states that the worst possible outcome evolving from a conflict is that we agree to disagree.

Managing conflict is a learned behavior. As we face the challenge to become more knowledgeable in the area of conflict management, there are some specific steps we can follow. When a given conflict presents itself, our first step is to decide if we are going to resolve it and, if so, how are we going to go about it? An important point to consider is that when two people are involved in a conflict, the two of them are the only persons who can resolve it.

Consider this conflict triangle:

If there is a conflict between person A and person B, normally they will discuss it with person C. It is reasonable for each of us to seek out someone with whom we feel comfortable about discussing a conflict we may have with another person. Eventually, person A must discuss the conflict with person B in order to resolve it. Person C would likely be the mediator between the other two.

Having looked at the possibility of resolving the conflict, several approaches are presented to us: (a) avoiding the conflict (withdrawal), (b) accommodating (smoothing), (c) compromising (sharing), (d) collaborating (problem solving) and (e) competing (forcing). We can make a decision to avoid a conflict at a given time for various reasons, but at some point it will need to be addressed. When we accommodate someone in a conflict, we simply give in to the other side. With the compromising approach, both sides gain and lose. When utilizing the competing or forcing approach, we must realize the possibility of losing completely. It is only when we collaborate about a conflict that it is possible to satisfy fully the needs of both sides.

Some behaviors that can help us become effective conflict managers are forming of alliances, willingness to compromise, learning the art of active delay, flexibility, exhibiting confidence and optimism, and being a likeable person. As supervisors, it is much to our advantage to know the art of conflict management and have the ability to teach our associates the techniques of conflict resolution. It is most exciting and rewarding to observe the growth and maturing of our associates in this very vital area of life.

IF YOU POINT A FINGER
AT
SOMEONE ELSE
YOU WILL BE POINTING
THREE
BACK AT YOURSELF

Chapter XVI

Quality Assurance

I really wish that I, personally, could make everyone aware of what quality assurance meant to me as a director of nursing. It is a management tool that can be very effective and enable each of us to stay in control of our facility. Quality assurance is a way of thinking. It is a way of turning problems into positive results. Remember that in the middle of difficulty lies opportunity. Once a problem is identified, it is half solved; quality assurance is a methodology utilized to consistently identify and solve problems.

Quality assurance is a systematic procedure for obtaining vital statistics about our facility. These are statistics that can help in dealing with patients, families, executive directors, associates and the general public. We can intelligently communicate the factual status of our facility to anyone. This kind of information is more readily accepted by the public than vague assurances that the facility is giving good care. For example, if you have proof that the facility has only one pressure ulcer, the sharing of this information with a family who is concerned about skin care, or the sharing of this information with the survey team as it arrives will give assurance that you are on top of things. It has been said that the only way to destroy false perceptions is to present the facts. A quality assurance system will routinely make these facts available to everyone.

The initial implementation of a quality assurance program/continuous quality improvement program requires organization and education, but once the program is established it is not a big job for anyone. It is a combination of several small ones that provide valuable information on an ongoing basis. By delegating certain responsibilities for the overall plan to several individuals within the facility, the plan can be implemented in a short period of time and the results will be of tremendous help to all concerned. We will all reap the benefits of our quality assurance efforts.

Quality patient care is the goal for which we are striving, the dream that we would like to realize. It has been said that the difference between a goal and a dream is that a goal has a plan. The difference in dreaming about quality patient care and producing that level of care is a good quality assurance plan fully implemented and thoughtfully carried through.

A good quality assurance plan permits management to know and monitor what is going on within the facility virtually at all times. Problems become situations to be discussed and reviewed; they arise as challenges to be met. A quality assurance plan provides for an environment in which each associate is constantly striving for perfection.

Associates learn to deal with actual results that are measured and quantified, not merely perceptions on how they may feel at any given time. These results can be shared with associates, with residents and family members, with state and federal quality assurance teams, and utilized in general in marketing campaigns and public relations efforts to demonstrate definite areas of strength.

Quality assurance programs will also allow the promotion of a sense of achievement among associates. It will encourage open communication, build self-esteem, promote training and education programs, and help with the management of goals. A good quality assurance program will present the opportunity to give quality patient care and make a commitment to excellence.

The first step in implementing a quality assurance program in a given facility is to select a quality assurance coordinator. The director of nursing, assistant director of nursing, an RN, LPN, or another individual in the facility may be appointed to that position. As soon as a qualified individual is in place, an educational process must begin. The quality assurance coordinator must be thoroughly knowledgeable of what quality assurance is and understand specific ways in which it can be implemented within the facility.

The next step is to further educate department heads, nursing supervisors and charge nurses as to the meaning of quality assurance and the importance of the program to each of them and their departments. Eventually, every associate in the facility will employ quality assurance problem-solving techniques to resolve difficulties at every level. This will be the time that all associates will bring forth their solutions instead of problems.

As soon as the personnel responsible for quality assurance functions have been identified and educated to their job duties, a committee must be appointed whose function will be to evaluate, agree upon and, finally, to implement the quality assurance plan in each facility. The challenge confronting us is to inspire our personnel to honestly seek in every endeavor to bring all problems to the surface, solve them, and to realize the importance of accountability in health care today. With these goals in mind, we sincerely covet the very best for quality assurance success in every facility.

As a quality assurance program is activated in our facility, we will discover how much it can assist us in progressively improving our facility to make it the best. The year 1989 was a great year for me as director of nursing. As an overall indicator of the quality of care, we achieved an occupancy rate of 99 percent. This occupancy rate assured me that our services were in demand and would continue to be needed. The 1989 survey results were very acceptable. Further training and concentration of each associates on his or her role in the operation of the facility would allow us to achieve our zero deficiency goal in 1990.

The training of new associates was a major undertaking and, may I add, a very successful one. Through facility efforts, we trained 36 new certified nursing technicians. We also had three of our associates attend and successfully complete LPN school and were successful in completing their state boards, thus becoming licensed practical nurses. We reactivated licenses for six RNs and/or LPNs and provided clinical training sites for 25 LPNs, RN-BSN students and 36 new certified nursing technicians. We were involved with East Tennessee State University and Vanderbilt University in research projects on Alzheimer's disease and drug utilization, respectively. We promoted nine associates to senior technician posts. This brought our total senior technician force to 18 in number.

In the dietary department, six associates completed their certification training requirements and became certified dietary technicians. The housekeeping department had five certified housekeeping technicians. Our dietary supervisor successfully completed the requirements, tested and became a certified dietary manager.

We had 27 associates who completed over three years of service with the facility and, of those, nine had completed over five years of service. Ten of our associates had a perfect work attendance record during 1989. I was honored by the Tennessee Health Care Association by being named the Outstanding Director of Nursing of the Year in Tennessee for 1989. These are just some of the accomplishments we are proud to have achieved.

The quality assurance program in the facility allowed us to continuously identify trends and priorities, thus allowing us to continuously improve our quality of care for our residents who are our highest priority. This process also allows for a continuous quality improvement focus which produces a very proud team of associates.

Absenteeism   GOAL = 2%

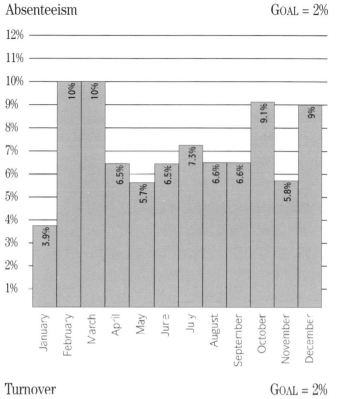

Turnover   GOAL = 2%

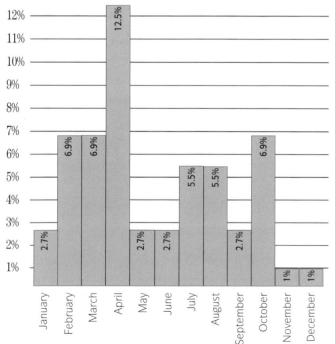

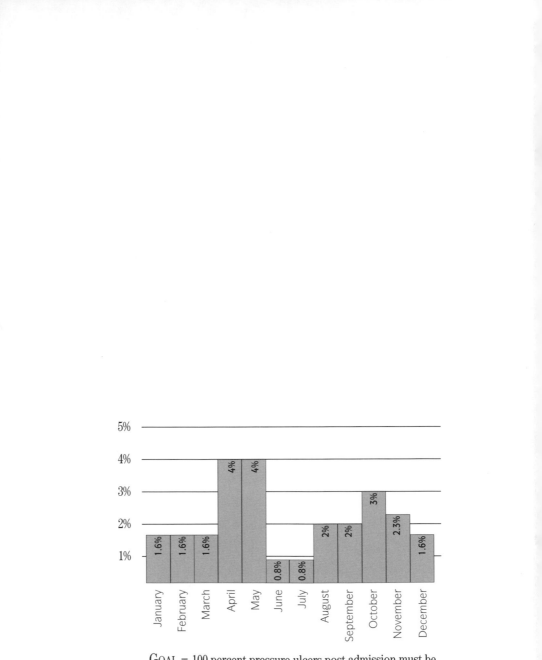

GOAL = 100 percent pressure ulcers post admission must be identified and healed at a Stage I.

The national average of nosocomial
infections in nursing facilities is five to ten percent.
The goal is to maintain that average. Monitoring
infections on a daily and monthly basis, reviewing
identified problems and implementing plans to
improve infection control rates will assist in
maintaining an acceptable rate.

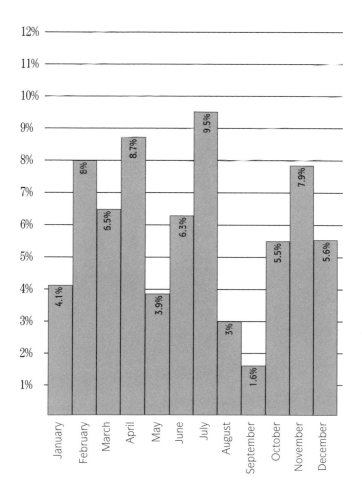

Poly-pharmacy (or the over-prescribing of medications) has garnered much publicity over the past few years. This is recognized as a potential problem among the elderly. We must pursue a very aggressive drug utilization and monitoring program. The national average is six separate prescriptions per patient per day in a nursing home.

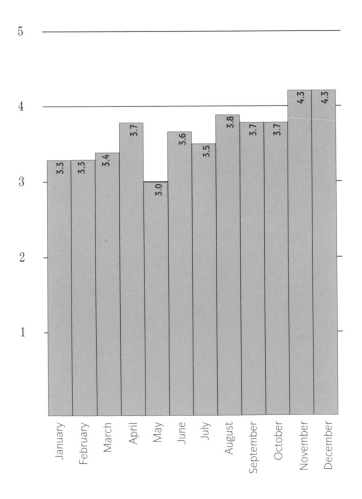

Weight loss is a chronic problem among the elderly. The ideal body weight of a patient is based upon his or her height and wrist measurements. A formula is then applied to these measurements to determine the patient's ideal body weight. Please note that ideal body weights do not take into consideration a patient's past weight history, lifestyle or eating habits. For instance, a patient's ideal body weight (based on this formula) may be 105 pounds; however, the patient may never have weighed more than 90 pounds in his/her entire life.

Also worthy of note is the fact that certain chronic diseases cause a weight loss. An important point to remember is that an awareness of and a continuous evaluation of underweight patients will help to determine what can be done to increase that weight if at all possible.

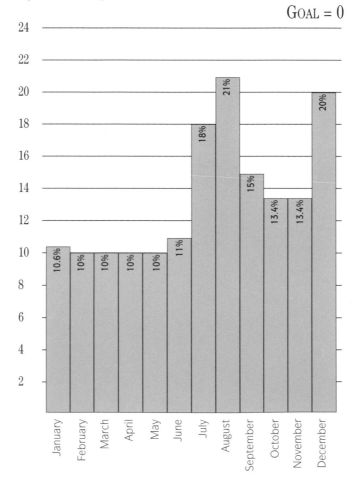

GOAL = 0

Residents who are 10% or more under their ideal body weight.

Graphs may also be utilized to visualize residents who have been identified in the other key weight loss areas.

Incidents are defined as any unusual occurrence. These reports give the Quality Assurance Committee the opportunity to spot potential problem areas, times of day, shifts, etc. The chart below shows the total percentage of incidents during a given year.

We can never guarantee that we will not have incidents in our facilities, but we can be in control of the incidents that do occur.

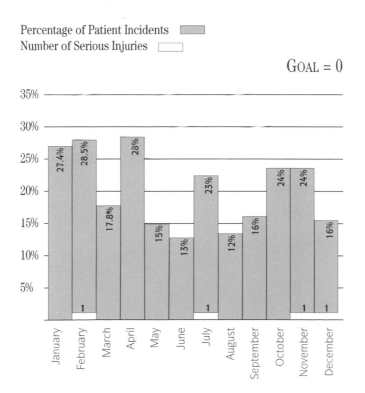

Percentage of Patient Incidents
Number of Serious Injuries

GOAL = 0

Dehydration is simply the loss of fluids from the body. Caused by a lack of adequate fluid intake or retention, which results from various illnesses or conditions, it is a serious problem among the elderly. The graph below depicts the number of patients diagnosed with dehydration over a one-year period of time.

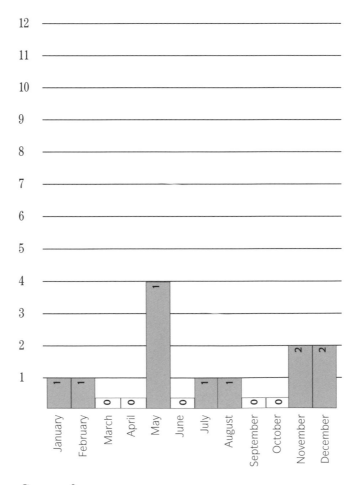

GOAL = 0

Antipsychotic medications are commonly used to alter behavior(s). They are used extensively among the elderly to treat dementia and are effective in altering the undesirable and sometimes dangerous behaviors. Although this is a valid method of treating such illnesses, we are sensitive to the possibility of the overuse of these types of medications. The "Drug Reduction Program" is a method of ensuring that every patient prescribed these medications is very closely monitored and that these medications are given for a valid medical reason. Through this program, one can be successful in eliminating and/or decreasing the use of these medications.

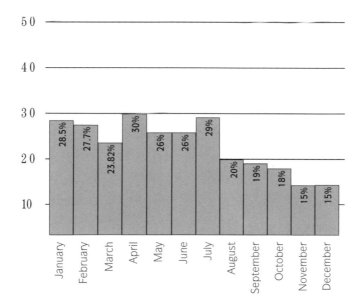

IT IS YOUR ATTITUDE
NOT
YOUR APTITUDE
THAT DETERMINES
YOUR ALTITUDE IN LIFE

Chapter XVII

Caring Enough to Make a Difference

All people need to love and be loved. We all care about others and are cared for by others. This relationship is a valuable part of our lives. In a fast-paced society such as ours, how do we maintain a caring mental attitude? How can we comfort and assure those around us that they will always be cared about and cared for? How can we make a difference in their lives? What does it mean to care enough to make a difference?

We realize that the long-term care field is a young industry. That being true, we realize that many of the concerns and challenges we presently face have never before been present. "Caring enough to make a difference" can be more clearly defined as we review some very important components of that concept.

In my mind, the term, caring, will become more active if we perceive it as commitment. Caring about someone gives rise to commitment on my part to develop a quality relationship. Commitment implies that I will be persistent and determined to accomplish that which is difficult and seemingly impossible. In the face of difficult situations in our lives, we often are tempted to walk away, to be overwhelmed and give up as the issues expand.

It is important to remember that everyone, without exception, encounters these challenges. The difference between success and failure is not whether or not we have made mistakes, but the way in which we have reacted to those mistakes. Caring and commitment dictate that I will not view any situation as a brick wall that I cannot get over, under, around or through, but each situation will be considered a challenge and a learning experience.

The word, education, comes to mind as I think of our industry and the challenges we face. We are progressing in our realization of the need for education among our personnel. The federal requirements for the training of nursing assistants is evidence of this progression. As directors of nursing, it becomes our responsibility, actually a very exciting challenge, to determine and make provision for the educational needs of the professionals under our supervision.

As we review the patient care indicators of such issues as infection rates, incident reports, weight control, pressure ulcers, etc., in our facility, we reflect upon our priority issues. What type of educational program will produce the highest quality of care for our residents? I will always contend that our associates desire to do a good job and it is our privilege and responsibility to make it possible for them to acquire the knowledge and skills required to attain the excellence for which we strive.

As we advance in commitment and educational procedure, we move to the process of building a teamwork structure. I was taught team nursing from the beginning of my career. There is no room for a hierarchy in nursing or in the entire health care profession. No one person is superior to another. Each person must be respected in his/her position—respect fosters respect. If I show respect for you, then you in turn are more likely to respect me. Every person is important in the provision of quality care for the resident. The attitude of servanthood becomes very valuable in our industry. How can we serve one another as well as our residents? Service can be evidenced in the form of actually assisting in a given task or in the areas of supporting, encouraging, teaching and being willing to learn from each other.

Management becomes a challenge to us as we begin to build our team and philosophy of management. We must identify the tools to be used in managing our department. Good management doesn't just happen—it is an art and a science. The manager must "direct the band," determine if anyone is off key, and teach the members how to fine-tune their skills to produce the highest quality of care–the ultimate outcome of our orchestrated efforts.

It is imperative that we develop an assessment process that will allow us to evaluate each situation objectively, consistently and impartially. We must keep our focus on the ultimate goal—quality care for our residents, our number one priority. Delegation of specific duties to others as well as accepting accountability for the outcome is part of our job as supervisor. Including others on our team should be a positive feature of our management style. For example, if I chose to appoint an LPN charge nurse to the position of infection control coordinator, she should perceive that as an honorable position and assist with a sense of pride in the management of the entire facility. This is an attitude we seek to instill in our staff as we discuss a management philosophy and build our management team.

My mission and purpose in life is to do everything within my power to see that elderly people in this country are well cared for and cared about; to see that the health care providers are well trained and proud to accept the responsibility for the provision of excellent care for the frail elderly of this country.

ASK YOURSELF THIS
QUESTION:
WHAT CAN "I" DO
TO MAKE
A DIFFERENCE?

CODE OF ETHICS

LOVE

Give love and you'll receive it.

CARE

Provide care for residents and staff to make a homelike atmosphere.

CONCERN

Concern for the facility 24 hours a day.

ATTENDANCE

Everyone working for perfect attendance. If we're not at work we can't do our jobs.

ATTITUDE

Counts 100 percent; our goal—to increase positive attitudes in the facility and community.

APPEARANCE

If you look good, you'll feel good.

TEAMWORK

Every shift, department and supervisor working together as a team.

PATIENT RIGHTS

Patients are first priority. Provide the best quality care.

THINK POSITIVE

Always think positive (a problem isn't the problem, it's the attitude about the problem.)

INVOLVEMENT	More involvement to better working relations; associate group activities—better working conditions.
FAMILY	Always be understanding toward family members.
HEALTH	Taking care of ourselves to take care of our residents.
RESPECT	Show respect for residents, family members and fellow associates.
GOALS	Set goals to better patient care and ourselves. Put God in our lives for guidance; with God all things are possible.
EMOTIONAL SUPPORT	Support each other in new ideas for bettering our facility.
SMILE	Always smile—it's contagious.
SUCCESS	If at first you don't succeed, try, try again.
COMMUNICATION	Let your fellow associates know what's going on, especially during shift change.
EAGERNESS	To work hard to make the facility the best.

PRIDE	Be proud of our jobs and take pride in everything we do.
RESPONSIBILITY	Carry through our responsibility; perform to the best of our ability.
IMPRESSION	First impressions are lasting impressions.
SENIOR TECHNICIANS	Work together as a team, not as individuals; uphold our positions to better ourselves for the benefit of our residents and the facility.

Senior Technicians Life Care Center of Erwin 1989

INDEX OF MEDICAL TERMS
FROM DORLAND'S MEDICAL DICTIONARY, 24TH ED.
AND THE MERCK MANUAL, 15TH ED.

agnosia
inability to recognize the import of sensory impressions - the inability to name things or people.

anosmia
absence of the sense of smell

anticoagulant
1) acting to prevent the clotting of blood
2) any substance which suppresses, delays or nullifies blood coagulation.

apraxia
loss of ability to carry out familiar purposeful movements in the absence of motor or sensory impairment, especially inability to use objects correctly (example - the inability to utilize the hand and arm to feed oneself).

dyskinesia
impairment of the power of voluntary movement. *Tardive dyskinesia* is characterized by choreiform movements of the buccal-lingual-fascial muscles, less commonly the extremities. Tardive dyskinesia may be caused by high doses of phenothiazines given over a long period of time (example - shaking of the hands as a side effect to antipsychotic drug utilization).

dystonia
impairment of muscular tonus.

extrapyramidal
functional, rather than anatomical, unit comprising the nuclei and fibers (excluding those of the pyramidal tract) involved in motor activities.

oculogyration
movement of the eye about the anteroposterior axis.

opisthotonos
a form of spasm in which the head and heels are bent backward and the body is bowed forward.

subcutaneous
beneath the skin.